Color Atlas of

SCLERITIS

Peter G Watson
MA MB B Chir FRCS FRCophth DO
Consultant Ophthalmic Surgeon
Head of Department of Ophthalmology
Addenbrooke's Hospital
University of Cambridge, Cambridge
Consultant Ophthalmic Surgeon
Moorfield's Eye Hospital
London

Joseph M Ortiz
MD FRCophth
Associate Clinical Professor of Surgery (Ophthalmology)
Cooper Hospital
University of Medicine and Dentistry of New Jersey
Camden, New Jersey
USA

Mosby-Wolfe

London Baltimore Bogotá Boston Buenos Aires Caracas Carlsbad, CA Chicago Madrid Mexico City Milan Naples, FL New York Philadelphia St. Louis Sydney Tokyo Toronto Wiesbaden

Copyright © 1995 Times Mirror International Publishers Limited

Published in 1995 by Mosby-Wolfe, an imprint of Times Mirror International Publishers Limited

Printed by Grafos S. A. Arte sobre papel, Barcelona, Spain.

ISBN 0 723 41753 9

For full details of all Times Mirror International Publishers Limited titles, please write to Times Mirror International Publishers Limited, Lynton House, 7–12 Tavistock Square, London WC1H 9LB, England.

A CIP catalogue record for this book is available from the British Library.

Library of Congress Cataloging-in-Publication Data applied for.

Project Manager:	Linda Kull
Developmental Editor:	Lucy Hamilton
Cover Design:	Lara Last
Production:	Mike Heath
Index:	Nina Boyd
Publisher:	Geoff Greenwood

Contents

Preface

This is an atlas, not a textbook, and therefore does not dwell on the underlying pathology. Its purpose is to enable the clinician to distinguish between the various manifestations of scleritis and episcleritis in order that appropriate therapy can be given. It is a sad fact that severe scleral disease is often left untreated, or allowed to continue unchecked until the patient's eyesight is affected, sometimes irreversibly. It is also true that, because the severity of the pain is apparently disproportionate to the visible physical signs, the patient's complaints are often ignored. Although scleritis is an unusual condition, its effect on the patient is so profound and it is so destructive to vision, that it is important that all ophthalmologists have a precise knowledge of the manifestations of the condition together with a clear understanding of the way in which each variety should be treated. This will ensure that those who need it are given adequate and effective treatment, and that those who do not require treatment are not given potentially toxic and dangerous therapy.

Throughout this atlas free use has been made of anterior segment fluorescein angiography to illustrate the underlying pathological process. Although extremely valuable when there is doubt as to the prognosis, the majority of patients with episcleral and scleral disease can be managed without it, provided that high magnification and red-free light are used during slit-lamp examination. However, B-scan ultrasound is essential to the diagnosis of posterior scleritis. If in doubt, this investigation must always be used.

Peter G. Watson
Joseph M Ortiz

Acknowledgements

We would like to thank the Departments of Medical Illustration at Moorfield's Eye Hospital, London, and Addenbrooke's Hospital, Cambridge for the care and attention to detail which has allowed the reproduction of the clinical photographs and angiograms.

We are grateful to Terry Tarrant for his exquisite and accurate drawings and to *Ophthalmology* for permission to reproduce them (**3.1–3.4**). We are also grateful to Mr Paul in Wolverhampton for permission to use the A- and B-scan ultrasounds (**5.72–5.80**) and to the *British Journal of Ophthalmology* and *Eye* for permission to reproduce the diagrams **2.2–2.4**.

The method of low-dosage fluorescein angiography is that developed by Dr Paul Meyer at Addenbrooke's Hospital, Cambridge and we would like to thank him for all the advice and help he has given us.

Bibliography

Foster, C.S., Sainz de la Maza, M. *The Sclera*. Springer–Verlag. New York, London, 1993.

Meyer, P. Low-dose fluorescein angiography patterns of blood flow in episcleral vessels studied by low-dose flourescein video angiography. *Eye* 2:533 1988.

Watson, P.G., Hazleman, B.L. *The Sclera and Systemic Disorders*. WB Saunders. London, Philadelphia, 1976.

1.
Introduction

It might be thought that episcleritis and scleritis, which are an inflammation of two very easily visible tissues, should be easy to diagnose and, because of the accessibility to local medication, easy to treat. Unfortunately, this is not the case. It is, for instance, notoriously difficult to be certain that the sclera is involved under the inflamed overlying tissues. It is even more difficult to diagnose inflammation of the posterior sclera when there are no visible signs in the retina or choroid and all that the patient is complaining of is loss of vision; for, although severe pain is usually a feature of posterior scleritis, the condition can occur without any pain at all.

In order to understand the techniques used in the diagnosis and differential diagnosis of episcleritis and scleritis, it is important to be clear about the normal anatomy of the tissues which become inflamed and their blood supply (**1.1**), because the first manifestations of both potentially serious life-threatening systemic disease and various forms of scleritis are seen through changes in the episclera and ocular vasculature.

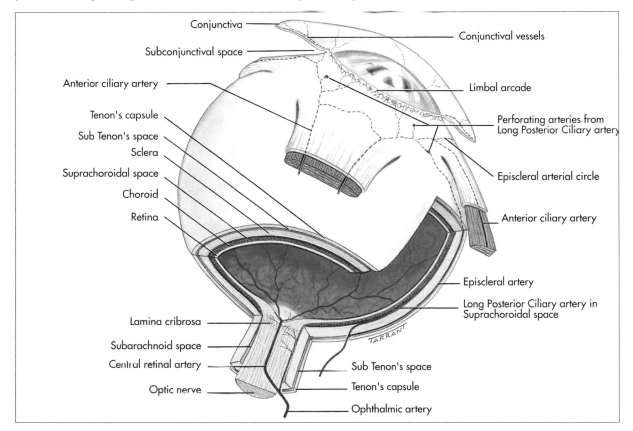

1.1 The sclera is completely covered with a fascial sheath (episclera) which adheres to the underlying tissue and a mobile superficial layer (Tenon's capsule). This allows the eye to move freely at all times. Tenon's capsule contains the episcleral blood vessels. Anteriorly it lies between the conjunctiva and the underlying sclera to which it is attached by fibrous bands. Posteriorly it is continuous with the muscular sheath, extends backwards to cover the whole of the globe and merges with the optic nerve sheath behind the eye. It is perforated by the ciliary vessels and nerves and the vortex veins.

2.
Surgical and Vascular Anatomy of the Sclera

Although not absolutely justified, it is convenient to think of the eye as an exposed ball-and-socket joint without articular cartilage and slightly modified for seeing. In man, the sclera consists of collagen fibrils of various sizes together with some elastic tissue at the equator, disc and limbus. The sclera derives its nutrition from the choroidal vasculature deep to it and the episclera which is attached to the underlying sclera by fibrous bands. The episclera is immobile whereas Tenon's capsule (fascia bulbi) is easily moved. Tenon's capsule, which contains the episcleral plexus of vessels, ensheaths the muscles and thickens in places to form the check ligaments and the ligament of Lockwood. Superficial to Tenon's capsule is the conjunctiva, the vessels of which anastomose with the episcleral vasculature at the limbus. The capsule is freely mobile but is attached to the underlying episclera by fibrous strands. Observation of these various layers is vital to the determination of the depth and extent of the inflammatory process in episcleral and scleral disease. This is best achieved by direct observation with the naked eye, preferably in daylight before using different magnifications on the slit lamp. The changes in the vasculature are confirmed by the use of red-free light (**2.1**).

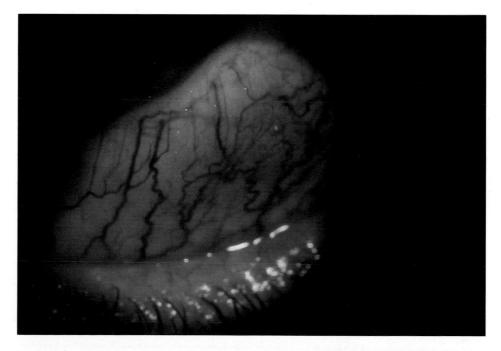

2.1 Red-free light examination. The green filter provided on all slit lamps should always be used to examine patients with suspected scleral disease. Blood vessels appear black in this light and transudates or clumps of lymphocytes appear yellow.

Red-free light examination will determine:

- Which part of the vascular tree is most dilated in the inflammatory response – the conjunctiva, or the episcleral or scleral vascular plexus.
- The patency of the vessels in each of the various layers.
- The rate of flow in patent vessels and the presence of re-routing of blood through other channels.
- Whether there are any areas of vaso-occlusion, non-perfusion or vaso-obliteration (this may have to be confirmed by angiography).
- Which areas are infiltrated and whether there is any swelling of tissues involved.
- Whether there are sites of vascular leakage into the cornea at the limbus.
- Whether there are any signs of necrosis or destruction.

It is of great importance to look for each of these features when examining patients with scleral inflammation, otherwise, not only will mistakes happen but vital clues as to the progression or regression of the disease will be missed.

It has always been a puzzle as to why scleral inflammation tends to start in the upper temporal and upper nasal quadrants of the sclera. Bearing in mind that scleritis often occurs in patients with connective tissue disease and that it is often associated with the vasculitic phase of these diseases, it seemed possible that the flow patterns in the vessels might provide the clues.

Meyer has shown, using anterior segment video angiography and haemoglobin imaging techniques, that there are regions in-between the major vessels in which there is periodically no flow of blood at all in the arteries, just a to-and-fro oscillation of blood within the vessels. It is here that the inflammation starts, suggesting that the poor flow may allow the initiation of the autoimmune response which is so characteristic of scleral disease.

In the course of his studies Meyer concluded that there are two major coronal circulations, and two sagittal circulations which meet, not as usual, through a capillary network and venous return, but as end-to-end arterial anastomoses with a common venous drainage (**2.2**). The reason for this is uncertain but it is probably a mechanism which ensures that the arterial blood supply of the anterior segment remains constant whichever way the eye is rotated. It is possible to examine the anterior part of this circulation in detail on the slit lamp and with various imaging techniques.

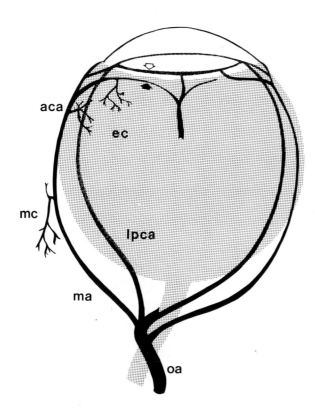

2.2 Arterial communications in the anterior segment of the eye. There are two arterial circulations in both the sagittal and coronal planes. The arterial ring inside the eye comes from the long posterior ciliary arteries and includes the major circle of the iris. The ring on the outside derives from the anterior ciliary arteries and the episcleral arterial circle. All these arteries communicate with each other. (Courtesy of Paul Meyer, Cambridge.)

Arterial communications in the anterior segment of the globe:

open arrow	intraocular arterial circle (major circle of iris)
closed arrow	extraocular arterial circle (anterior episcleral arterial circle)
oa	ophthalmic artery
ma	artery of rectus muscle
aca	anterior ciliary arteries (joined by episcleral arterial circle)
lpca	long posterior ciliary artery
ec	episcleral capillaries
mc	muscular capillaries

note: ma + aca + scleral perforator + lpca form a sagittal arterial ring.

In order to understand the pathology it is important to be able to distinguish the various components of the circulation (**2.2–2.4**). Blood enters the superficial vascular plexuses from the conjunctival vessels at the limbus (in vessels derived from the external carotid artery), from the anterior ciliary arteries anterior and adjacent to the rectus muscles (two to each except the lateral rectus) and, more surprisingly, from the long posterior ciliary arteries via the perforating vessels in the anterior sclera. Blood usually flows in these vessels from inside to the outside of the eye. Having perforated the sclera the arteries anastomose with those of the anterior ciliary circulation to form the episcleral arterial circle which is usually incomplete in man but almost always joins the territory of one anterior ciliary circulation to the next. Branches from this circle pass backwards to form the capillary networks of the

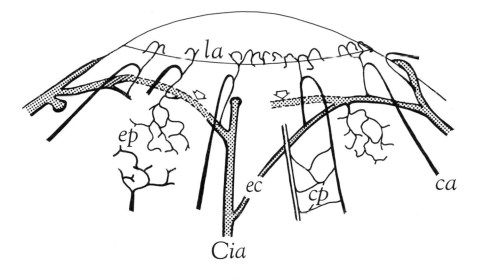

2.3 The arterial supply of the conjunctiva and episclera. (Courtesy of Paul Meyer, Cambridge.)

Cia	*anterior ciliary artery*
ec	*anterior episcleral arterial circle (deep component marked)*
ca	*conjunctival arteriole*
ep	*episcleral capillary plexus*
cp	*conjunctival capillary plexus*
la	*limbal arcades*

2.4 The circulation of the human limbus. In regions where blood from the anterior and posterior ciliary arteries meet there is no flow only oscillation of blood in the vessel. (Courtesy of Paul Meyer, Cambridge.)

The circulation of the human limbus

lpca	*long posterior ciliary artery*
aca	*anterior ciliary artery*
open arrow	*episcleral arterial circle*
closed arrow	*limbal venous circle*
ev	*episcleral collecting vein*

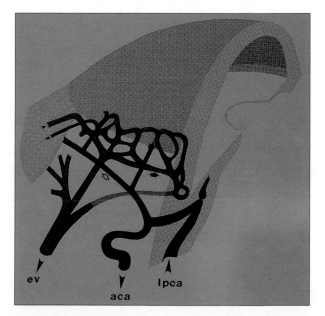

episclera and Tenon's capsule and forwards to form the limbal arcades. In the normal young individual the arteries tend to be tortuous, the capillary beds fill evenly and completely and the veins are straight. The limbal arcades are intact and completely regular. All these features can be easily seen on low dose anterior segment fluorescein angiography and none of the vessels leak until very late in the angiogram if at all (**2.5–2.14**).

Having understood the nature of the blood supply of the anterior segment, it becomes easier to understand the various clinical syndromes associated with inflammation of the anterior sclera. Using B-scan ultrasound it is possible to show that these syndromes occur in the posterior segment also. They are much more difficult to diagnose but the treatment options remain the same.

Normal anterior segment low dose fluorescein angiogram of the limbal circulation

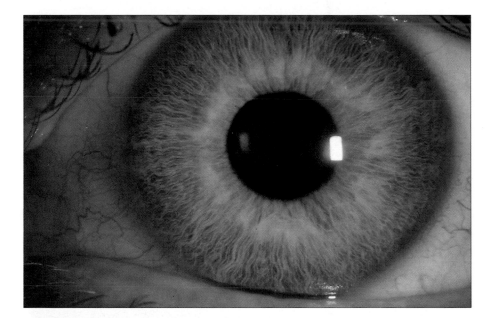

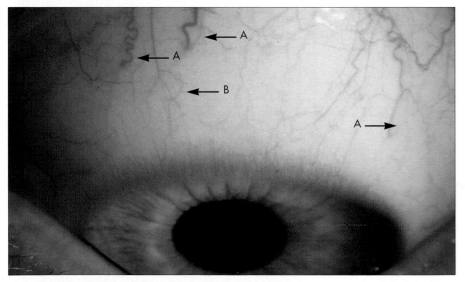

2.5, 2.6 The normal anterior segment. Several perforating vessels (A) can be seen. These are tortuous and are arterial. These vessels anastomose with the anterior ciliary arteries over the superior rectus muscle. Flow in these vessels may be in either direction. The area labelled (B) is shown in more detail in **2.7–2.14**.

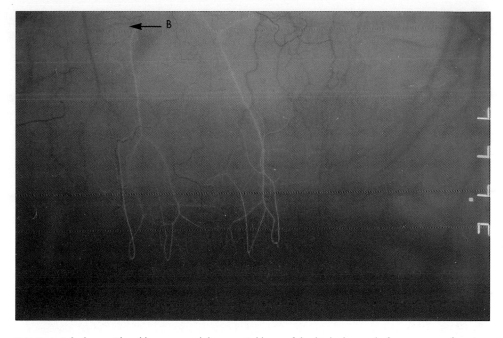

2.7 Arterial phase. Blood has entered the arterial loop of the limbal arcade from two perforating vessels.

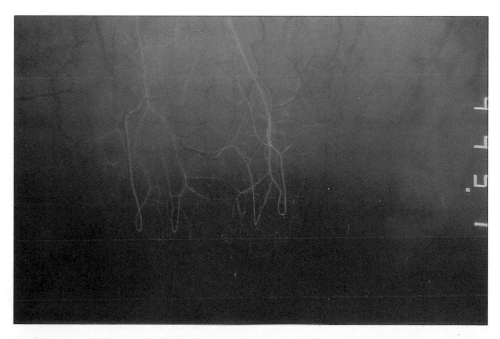

2.8 Late arterial phase. Blood which has entered the loop does not leak from the vessels. The arcade, which is absolutely regular, is formed by the joining of the two arteriolar loops near the tip of the arcade.

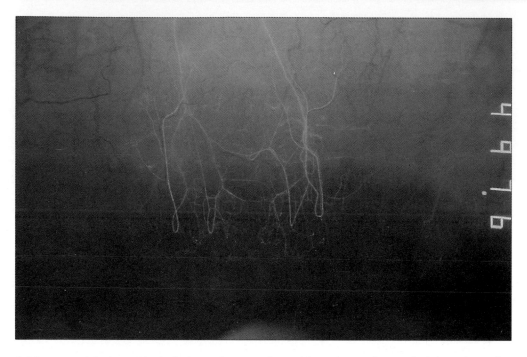

2.9 Late arterial phase. The limbal arcade is now formed from the two loops which have formed in two places. The capillary bed in between is now full.

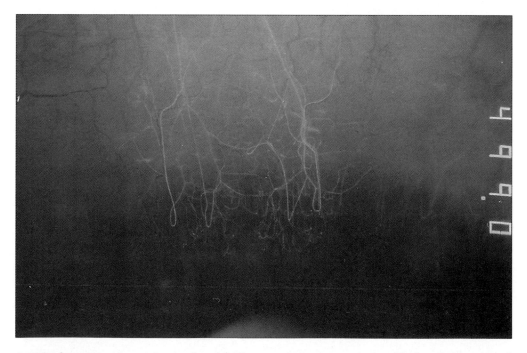

2.10 Early venous phase. The capillary bed between the two arterioles has filled and venous blood is being drained superficially to the episcleral veins. A further arterial loop is now contributing from one side. The capillaries derived from the largest vessels can be seen to extend beyond the arterial loops.

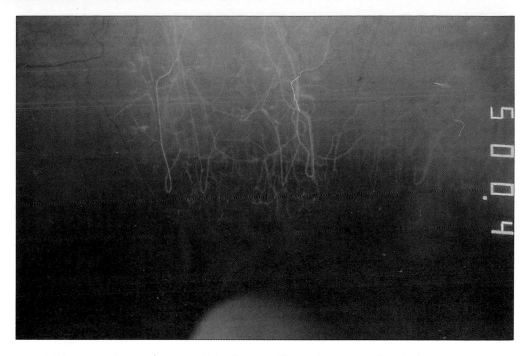

2.11 Mid-venous phase. The arterial blood is now filling adjacent capillary beds.

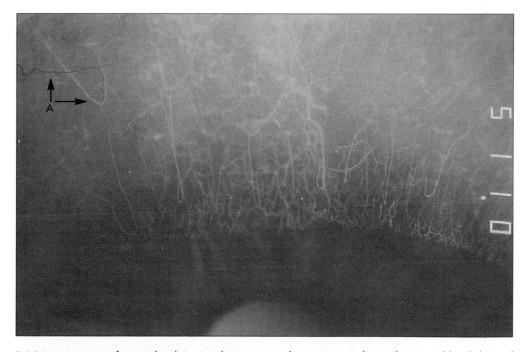

2.12 Late venous phase. Blood is now draining into the conjunctival vessels to join blood derived from the conjunctival arteries. Early leakage can be seen from these vessels. A peripheral loop (A) of the episcleral arterial circle can be seen. The filling of this vessel is transient and rapid (**2.14**).

2.13 Late venous phase. The limbal circulation is now complete, is regular and communicates with the neighbouring capillaries. There is now a contribution from the conjunctival vessels which can be seen to leak fluorescein.

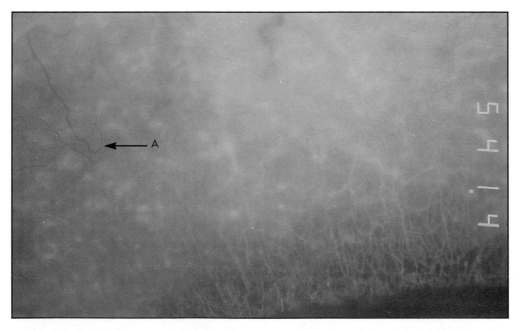

2.14 Late venous phase. There is marked conjunctival leakage. The episcleral circle (A) is non-fluorescent. Note that even at this very late stage the limbal capillaries still do not leak.

3.
Classification of Episcleritis and Scleritis

Clinically, inflammation which involves episclera and Tenon's capsule without underlying oedema of the sclera is termed episcleritis. The inflammation may be diffuse (simple episcleritis), in which it affects part or the whole of the outer covering, or it may become aggregated into nodules in which the exudate remains localized to one area (nodular episcleritis). The milder forms of scleritis follow a similar pattern, except that there is some involvement of the underlying sclera and the inflammation is more intense (**3.1–3.4**).

Necrotizing scleritis is quite different. In this condition the sclera and all its coats, often including the overlying conjunctiva, become involved in a destructive granulomatous process which if inadequately treated will lead to the destruction of the eye and the inevitable loss of vision. The object of all the investigations is to be sure that necrotizing scleritis is detected early and that the underlying systemic disease which is present in 70% of these patients is found and treated. One form of episcleritis or scleritis does not change to another. The disease found at presentation is the condition which will be present in all recurrences.

Episcleritis

Diffuse (Simple)
Nodular

Scleritis (May be anterior, posterior or both)

Diffuse
Nodular
Necrotizing   with inflammation
               without inflammation
               (scleromalacia perforans)

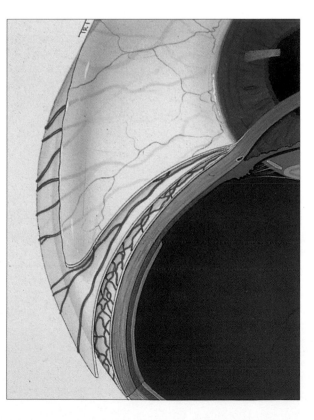

3.1 Diagram of the normal vascular arrangements. There is a layer of vessels on the surface of the sclera which contributes to its nutrition. A second layer occupies the Tenon's capsule (the superficial episcleral tissue), and also a further layer, derived from the external carotid circulation in the overlying conjunctiva.

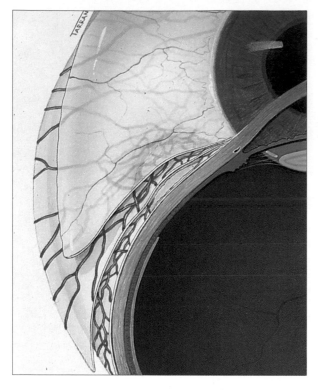

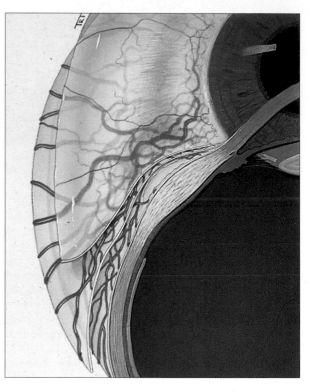

3.2 Episcleritis. In episcleritis the inflammation and infiltration of tissue is confined to the episcleral vasculature. The conjunctival vessels may or may not be congested.

3.3 Anterior scleritis. In anterior scleritis the sclera is swollen and infiltrated displacing all the vessels of the episclera forwards. The episcleral tissues are also swollen so attention must be given to observing the contour of the scleral surface. Depending on the severity of the inflammation the vessels of the episclera may be irregular or non-perfused and this may affect the limbal circulation.

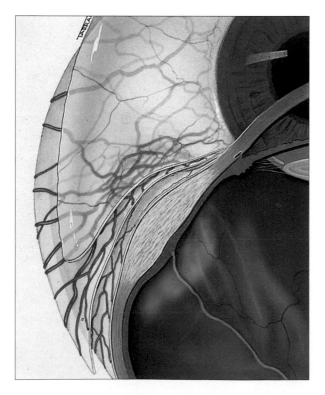

3.4 Posterior scleritis. Posterior scleritis can arise in the posterior segment alone but more commonly, as here, is an extension of the scleritis from the anterior segment. If severe this will cause sub-retinal transudation resulting in a non-rhegmatogenous retinal detachment.

4.
Episcleritis

There are two major types of episcleritis: simple or diffuse episcleritis and nodular episcleritis.

Our knowledge of the course and aetiology of simple episcleritis has advanced little since 1895 when it was accurately described by Fuchs as episcleritis periodica fugax, a transient periodic inflammation of the episclera. It is much more commonly seen in young women than men, is rarely uncomfortable and is never damaging to the eye. The appearance and the prickly sensation it produces do however cause considerable distress to some patients who demand some form of treatment. Unless the inflammation is very severe or prolonged, there is little point in undertaking any investigations, as these are almost universally negative. However, a careful history sometimes reveals a precipitating factor which if eliminated may be successful in preventing recurrences. If the attacks are prolonged beyond 21 days they should be investigated in the same way as for patients with scleritis, as many of these will be found to have some underlying systemic disorder.

Clinically, although the redness may be very intense, examination reveals that the inflammation is confined to the episcleral tissue (the conjunctival vessels remain normal or are only slightly dilated). There is no distortion of the vascular pattern, although rate of flow of blood through the vessels is increased and the vessels are more permeable (4.1–4.8). There is no discharge or pain, only discomfort.

In nodular episcleritis the vessels in one area of the episclera become much more permeable, allowing a localized aggregation of inflammatory cells and exudate (4.9–4.12). As in simple episcleritis there is no undue discomfort, and there is no discharge from the eye. A normal vascular pattern is maintained although the vessels in the area of the episcleral nodule are dilated, are freely permeable and the blood flows very rapidly through them. The underlying scleral tissue is not involved. Clinically the course is much the same as with simple episcleritis but because of the localized oedema the resolution tends to be slower. Only those with very persistent disease should be fully investigated.

Therapy

Episcleritis is a superficial disorder rarely associated with any systemic disease. It is self-limiting although recurrent and unless it causes acute discomfort requires no treatment. If treatment is necessary and non-steroidal anti-inflammatory agents are available for local use, one of these should be given. Local steroids will reduce the inflammatory response and increase the patient's comfort but should not be used on a continuing basis because they can induce glaucoma and cataract. Steroids do not change or shorten the course of the disease. Very occasionally if there is persistent and painful inflammation unresponsive to local therapy, or if local therapy is contra-indicated a systemic non-steroidal anti-inflammatory agent may have to be given. The most effective appears to be flurbiprofen 100 mg three times daily. This can be stopped as soon as the inflammation is suppressed.

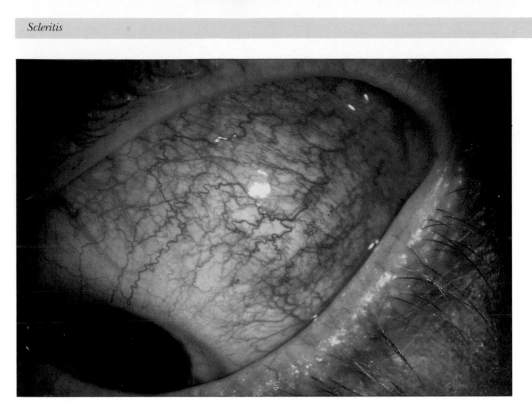

4.1 Simple episcleritis. The inflammation involves all the visible episclera. Although intensely congested the vascular pattern remains normal. The conjunctival vessels are slightly dilated, but the episcleral vessels are much more dilated.

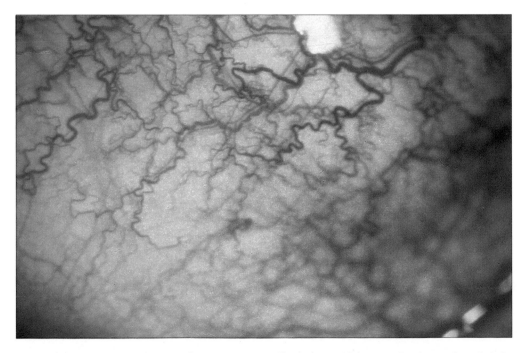

4.2 Simple episcleritis. This eye shows intensive inflammation of the episcleral vessels with little obvious oedema, although the vascular layers can be seen to have been separated.

4.3–4.5 Angiography in simple episcleritis. Fluorescein angiogram of **4.2**. The photographs of the angiogram are taken at 1 second intervals. The circulation time is extremely rapid. All the vessels fill and leak immediately but the vascular pattern is not disturbed.

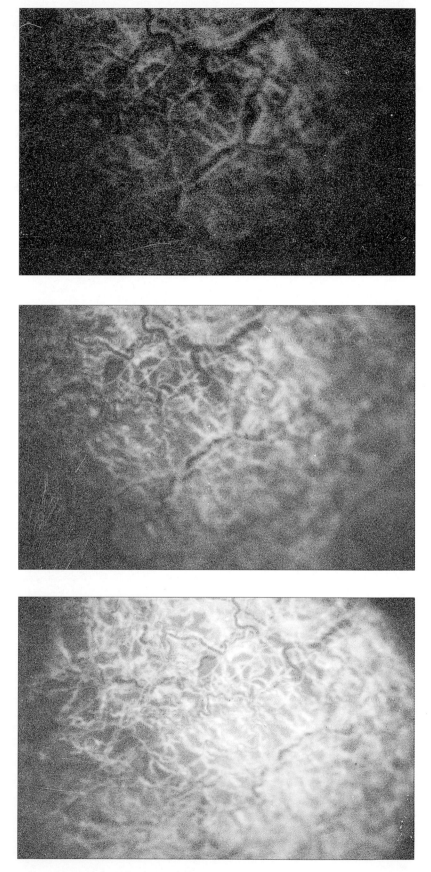

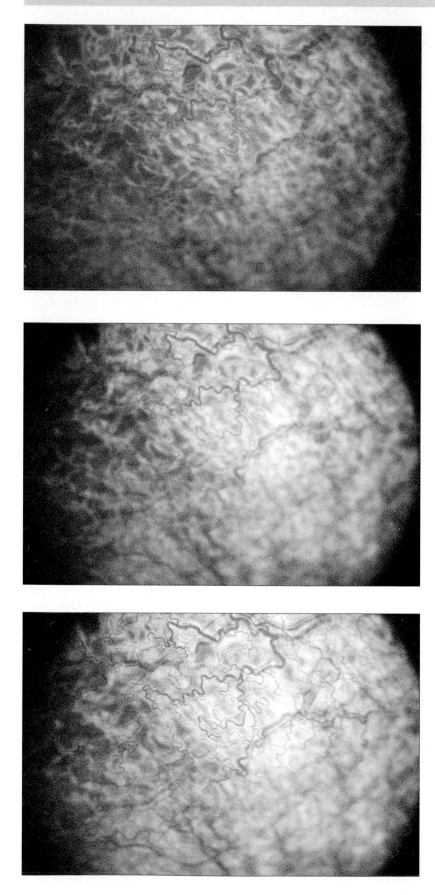

4.6–4.8 Angiography in simple episcleritis. After 4 sec (**4.6** upper), 5 sec (**4.7** middle) and 15 sec (**4.8** lower). At 15 sec (the timing of the early venous phase of the normal angiogram) the circulation is complete and there is diffuse leakage into the extravascular space.

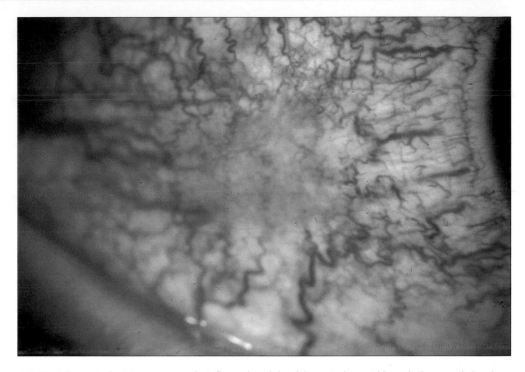

4.9 Nodular episcleritis. An intensely inflamed nodule of the episclera. Although the vessels leading to the site of the nodules are very congested, their normal arrangement is not disturbed.

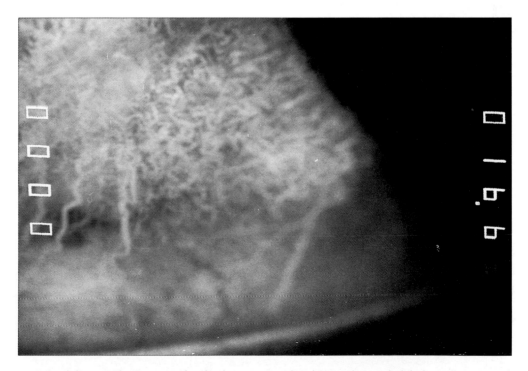

4.10 Nodular episcleritis. Here the dye has appeared in the circulation slightly later than normal (14 sec), but there is immediate leakage from both arterioles and capillaries at the site of the nodule.

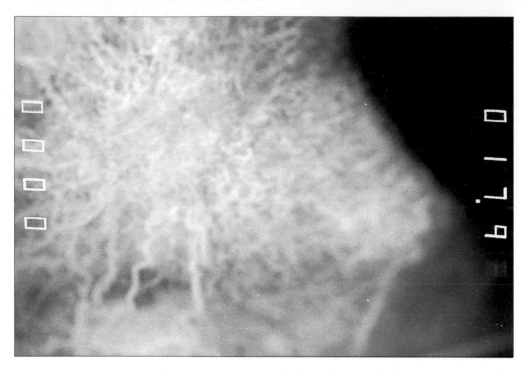

4.11 Nodular episcleritis. After another 1.3 sec, the leakage has extended to the veins and to the limbal arcades.

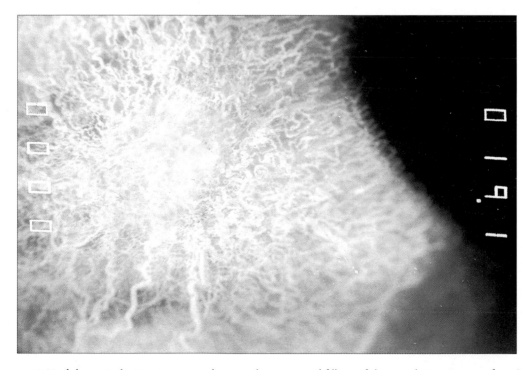

4.12 Nodular episcleritis. Angiography reveals very rapid filling of the circulation (2.5 sec from the first appearance of the dye) and immediate leakage into the nodule. The limbal phase is complete, its pattern is not disturbed and these vessels do not leak dye.

5.
Scleritis

Scleritis, be it anterior or posterior, is an extremely painful disease which tends to be referred to the temple and face rather than be seated in the eye itself. Characteristically, it wakes the patient during the night; it is usually this that brings the patient for treatment.

However, scleritis can occur without pain, particularly in scleromalacia perforans and in some patients with posterior scleritis. It is therefore important to consider posterior scleritis as a diagnosis when faced with patients with loss of vision, a slightly swollen disc or exudative retinal detachments.

Scleritis, like episcleritis, is a recurrent condition and is usually bilateral even though the onset, which is usually insidious, may be delayed in the second eye for several years. The disease is almost always self-limiting, so that, if adequate treatment can be given, sight-threatening changes can be prevented. It follows, therefore, that the correct early diagnosis is essential.

This is done by taking a careful history to ascertain: the type of onset; symptoms, such as the type of pain and its distribution; the presence of photophobia and watering of the eye; and symptoms suggestive of underlying connective tissue disease. If there is any doubt, the opinion of a rheumatologist or other interested physician should be sought. Routine investigation of the haemoglobin levels, a differential white cell count, erythrocyte sedimentation rate, 'C' reactive protein, serum uric acid, serology for syphilis and an immunological survey should be undertaken. The immunological survey should include immunoglobulin levels, the autoantibodies, Rheumatoid Factor (RhF), antinuclear antibodies (ANA) (DNA binding). If the physical signs suggest a systemic vasculitis, anti-nuclear cytoplasmic antibody tests (pANCA and cANCA) should be performed. These investigations will reveal the presence or absence of severe underlying systemic disease, which may not be apparent even on the most careful examination, so determining whether the patient is likely to need immunosuppressive therapy rather than treatment with anti-inflammatory agents.

Ocular examination has to be directed at deciding whether the sclera itself, rather than just the coats of the eye, is involved; and if so, whether this inflammatory process is leading, or is likely to lead, to destruction of that tissue and those around it. The presence of anterior scleritis can usually be deduced by physical examination, but the diagnosis of posterior scleritis is difficult because its presence can only be implied from its effect on the surrounding tissues. Even then, severe posterior scleritis may be present without any visible signs in the retina or choroid. It is only possible to examine the posterior sclera with B-scan ultrasonography, although the methods are not yet sophisticated enough to decide whether the choroid or sclera are involved together or separately. If B-scan ultrasonography is not available, CT scanning or MRI scanning with an orbital coil will identify the swollen tissue.

Anterior scleritis

Clinically, scleritis presents as a diffuse, nodular or necrotizing scleritis. It is very unusual for a condition to progress from one form to another, although some patients in the course of this disease will have a nodular attack on one occasion and a diffuse one on another, and the occasional person will develop necrosis within a large scleral nodule. Nodules can sometimes be multiple but each small nodule shows the same characteristics as the larger ones.

The diagnosis of anterior scleritis, which accounts for at least 75% of all patients with scleritis, depends on the observation that the sclera itself is involved in the inflammatory process. The overlying inflammation is much more intense than in episcleritis (**5.1**). This sometimes causes conjunctival chemosis (**5.2–5.5**), so in order to observe the contour of the underlying sclera it may be necessary to blanche the vessels using 10% phenylephrine drops. Having observed that the sclera is oedematous the next important decision is whether this lesion is destructive or potentially so. This requires careful examination of the vessels as scleritis is caused by a T-cell mediated granulomatous change accompanied by a vasculitis that is sometimes the primary lesion. Initially this appears to be a venulitis, the arterial tree becoming involved later (**5.6–5.12**). The vascular changes caused by the inflammation can be detected by anterior segment fluorescein angiography, as can the non-perfusion, vaso-obliteration and re-routing of blood which indicates the onset or presence of necrotizing scleritis.

Anterior uveitis accompanying scleritis is extremely rare and, if cells are present in the anterior or posterior chamber, this indicates either serious disease or the wrong diagnosis.

Diffuse anterior scleritis

Diffuse anterior scleritis is the most benign type of scleritis but it is also frequently misdiagnosed leading to unnecessary pain and discomfort in the patient and occasionally a permanent reduction in visual acuity.

The main differentiating feature from episcleritis is the intense pain, which radiates from the eye to the temple or into the face. The pain commonly wakes the patient in the early hours of the morning, gradually fading as the day progresses. The redness can be intense (**5.1**) and may be associated with chemosis of the conjunctiva (**5.2–5.5**), but more commonly there is a redness of the anterior segment. The condition is usually unilateral in each attack but may affect both eyes from time to time and is accompanied by some photophobia and watering which is worse if the pain is intense.

It is often difficult to tell whether the underlying sclera is swollen even after the superficial vessels have been blanched. If in doubt, the configuration of the vessels themselves should be examined with care. In episcleritis the vessels, although dilated, retain their normal pattern and the capillary nets are readily visible and patent. In scleritis, however, areas of capillary closure occur, and the venules leak and become partially or totally occluded (**5.6–5.12**). As a consequence the vascular pattern becomes distorted and abnormal. The easiest place to see these changes is the limbus, where the normally completely regular capillary arcade becomes distorted, irregular and degenerate. As these changes are permanent, an abnormality of this network suggests a current or old attack of scleral inflammation (**5.9–5.12**).

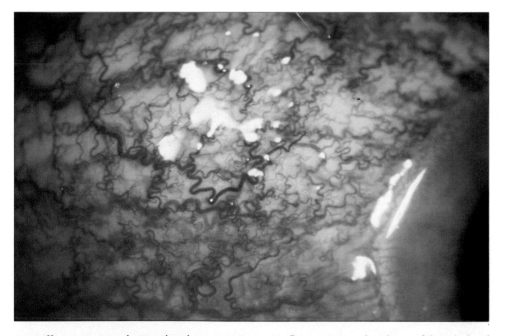

5.1 Diffuse anterior scleritis. This shows very intense inflammation and oedema of the whole of the anterior episclera with dilatation of both the conjunctival and deep episcleral vessels. The limbal arcades are dilated but not disrupted. To determine whether the sclera is swollen, phenylephrine 10% drops should be applied to blanche the superficial vessels and allow the sclera to be seen.

Diffuse anterior scleritis

5.2–5.5 *Intense chemosis in a patient with diffuse anterior scleritis who had no other known systemic disease.*

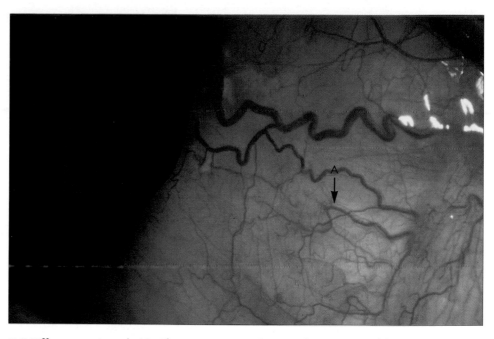

5.2 Diffuse anterior scleritis. There is intense oedema and congestion of the conjunctiva and episclera at the limbus. The arteries are large and prominent.

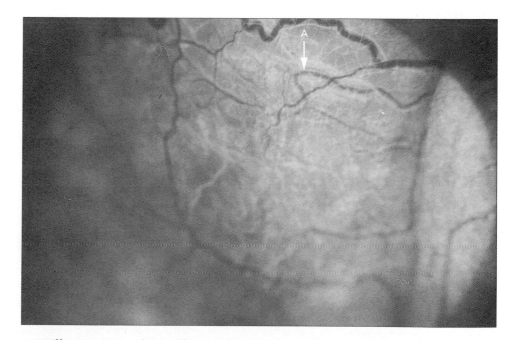

5.3 Diffuse anterior scleritis. Fluorescein angiogram of area of **5.2** (A). There is early and immediate leakage into the extravascular space. No blood is visible in the main vessels either, through obstruction to flow (possibly by thickening of the vascular wall). The fine arterioles show beading of the blood column, indicating a very sluggish blood flow or occlusion of the vessel.

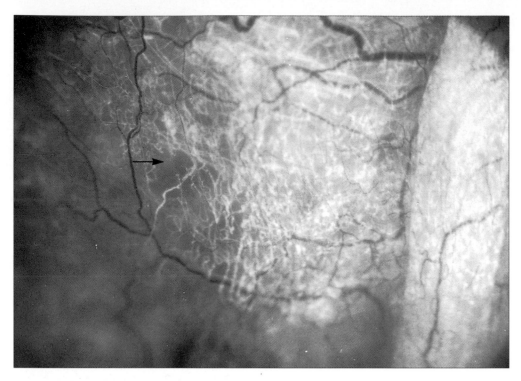

5.4 Diffuse anterior scleritis. Venular obstruction of some vessels with leakage points. Other vessels are dilated and there is an area of complete capillary 'drop out' (arrowed).

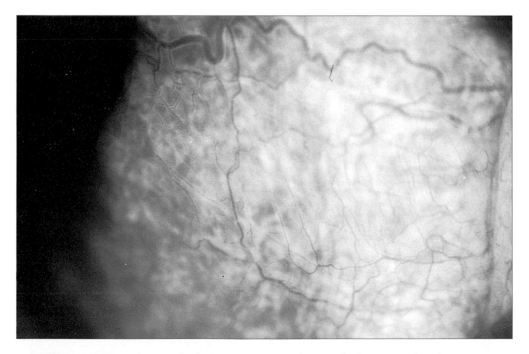

5.5 Diffuse anterior scleritis. The late angiogram with gross leakage into the chemotic area. Fluorescein staining can be seen at the periphery of the major vessels.

Diffuse anterior scleritis

5.6–5.12 Although the inflammation is less intense than that seen in 5.1–5.5, there is an area of oedema adjacent to the limbus (A) which has led to diffuse corneal infiltration by serum residues.

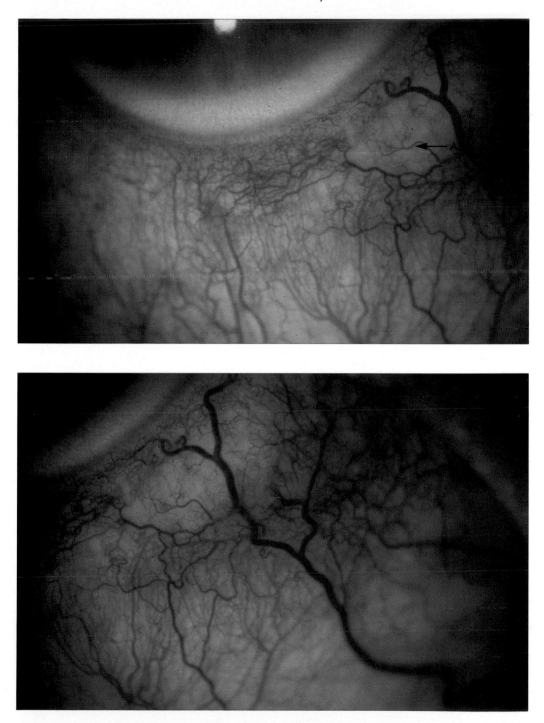

5.6, 5.7 Angiography revealed that the oedema is due to leakage from the deep scleral vessels (long posterior ciliary vessels). There is also an area of hypoperfusion of the superficial layers of the limbal episcleral and conjunctival vessels, i.e. the inflammatory response has been initiated in the deep tissues.

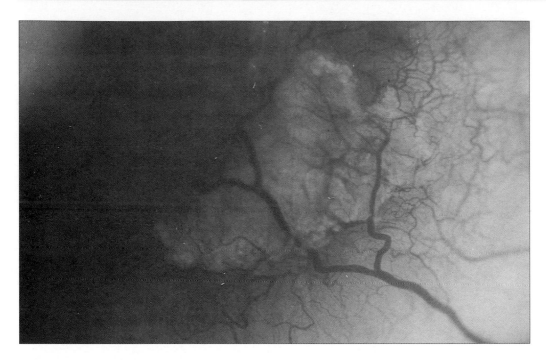

5.8 Diffuse anterior scleritis. Same patient as in **5.6**. Early arterial phase. Note that there is staining from leakage of the long posterior ciliary vessels which highlights the non-perfused superficial circulation. There is an area adjacent to the limbus where only very large vessels can be seen.

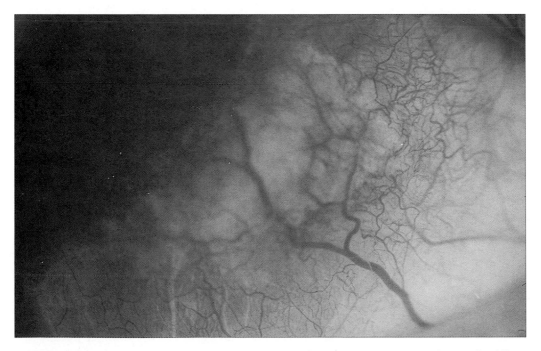

5.9 Diffuse anterior scleritis. Some vessels are being filled from the conjunctival circulation. The diffuse deep scleral leakage has increased.

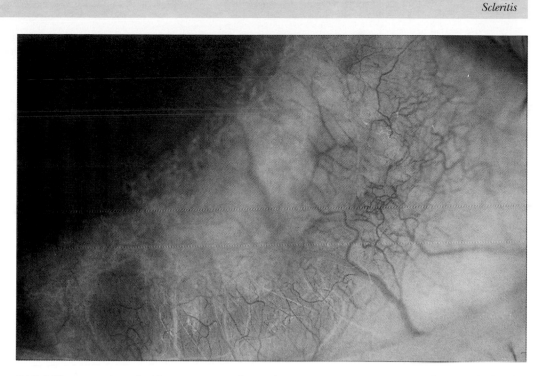

5.10 Diffuse anterior scleritis. Late venous phase of anterior segment angiogram also reveals that the limbal arcades are non-perfused at 6 o'clock, with another area of non-perfused vessels adjacent to it. Streaming can be observed in the veins leaving the oedematous area.

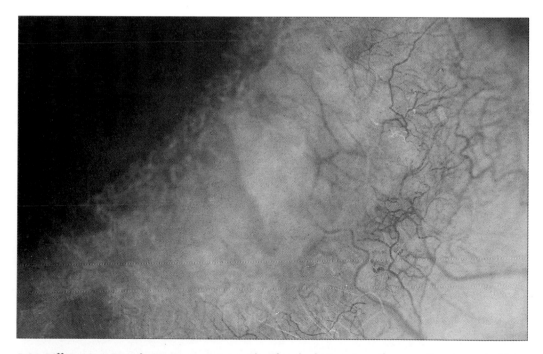

5.11 Diffuse anterior scleritis. Deep staining identifies the large areas of non-perfused vessels. Those capillaries that have some blood in them show beading, indicating an almost static circulation. The normal vascular pattern of both the episcleral vessels and the inferior limbal arcades has been lost.

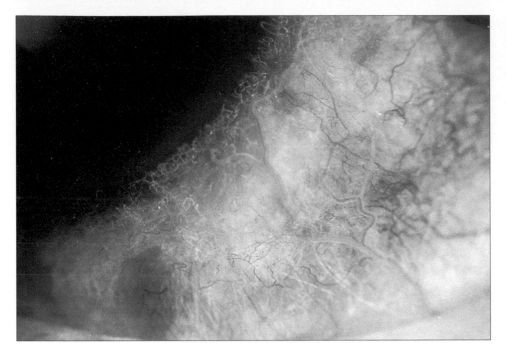

5.12 Diffuse anterior scleritis. A late photo taken to show the disruption of the limbal arcade and a very sluggish flow in some of the major vessels.

Nodular scleritis

Nodular scleritis is different from nodular episcleritis. Not only are the nodules fixed, but they are extremely painful and tender to the touch.

Nodular scleritis tends to be bilateral (**5.13–5.18**), although commonly only one eye is affected at a time. The nodules often recur at the same site and are accompanied by referred pain to the head, lacrimation and photophobia. They may be single or multiple. If the multiple nodules occur close to the limbus, they can be accompanied by sharp rises in intraocular pressure.

Many patients with nodular scleritis have no associated systemic disease, but some who are in the late extra-articular stages of rheumatoid arthritis can develop pain-

less scleral rheumatoid nodules (**5.19– 5.22**) which rarely require treatment and which fade spontaneously.

Biopsy or excision of scleral nodules is rarely justified and should only be done in exceptional circumstances. Small biopsies rarely reveal anything of value, apart from confirming the inflammatory process and the types of cells involved, although certain unusual diagnoses can be made. Large nodules are often full of liquid degenerative collagen. If left alone, the nodule will be replaced by fibrous tissue after treatment; but if it is removed, it will leave bare choroid. However, the large nodules in **5.13** were removed because the patient was unable to close her eyes properly. They were solid and the final result was good.

Nodular anterior scleritis

5.13–5.18 A 36-year-old female with no known systemic disease presented with gradual onset of bilateral nodular scleritis. Over a period of five years, both eyes periodically became intensely inflamed with intensive immediate deep leakage into the nodule (*5.14*), which is present even in the early arterial phase of the angiogram. Because the nodules remained between attacks and were persistently uncomfortable, they were excised, but the biopsy was unhelpful in establishing a diagnosis. Scleral nodules should not normally be excised, as they often contain degenerate liquid collagen which if released leaves the choroid exposed. Fortunately, these nodules were solid and the final result was good with no recurrence of the problem (*5.18*).

5.13 Right eye.

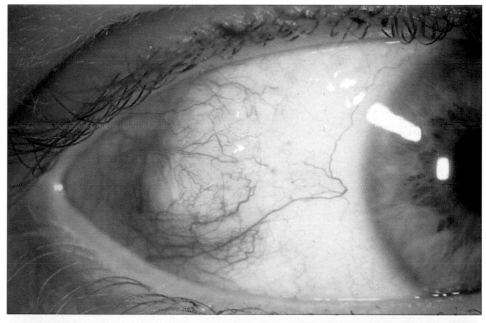

5.14 Left eye.

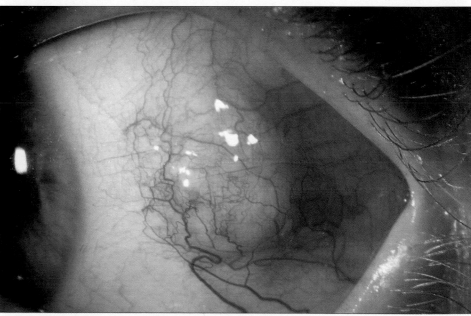

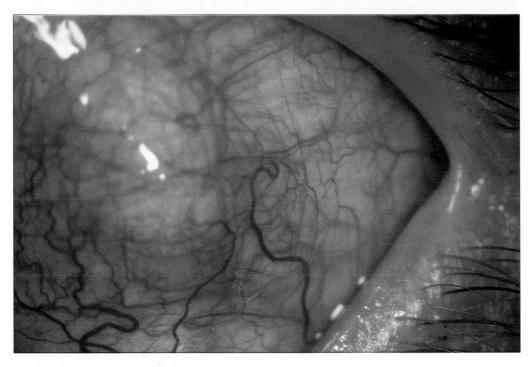

5.15 Nodular anterior scleritis. Infra-red photo of **5.14** showing the dilated capillary networks and abnormal vascular pattern on the corneal side of the nodule which is out of focus because of its large size. The vessels on and around the nodule are tortuous and abnormal.

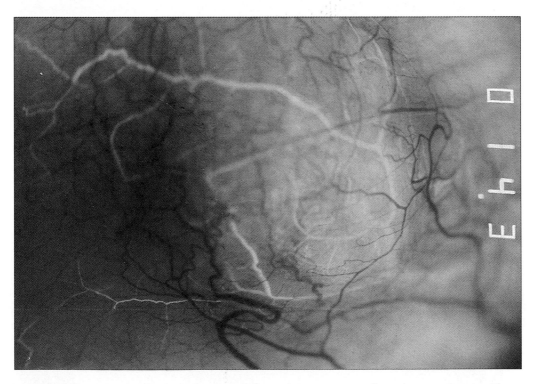

5.16 Nodular anterior scleritis. Early arterial phase anterior segment fluorescein angiogram. There is beading and sluggish flow in the early arterial phase, with no immediate leakage into the nodule (cf **4.7–4.12**).

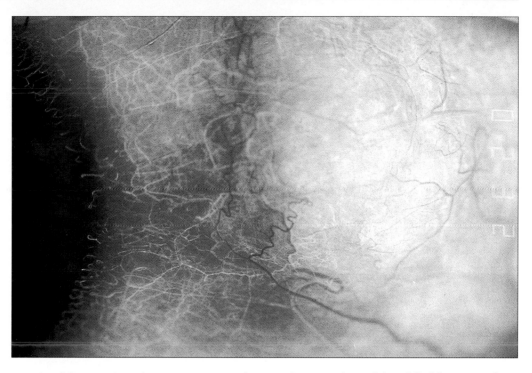

5.17 Nodular anterior scleritis. Late venous phase. At this stage the nodule is full of fluorescein from leaking vessels. The limbal and episcleral circulation is sluggish with 'cattle trucking'. The limbal arcades are disrupted between 2 and 4 o'clock, with a few new vessel fronds beginning to form.

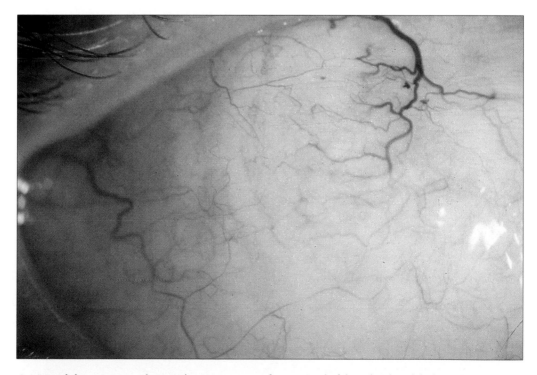

5.18 Nodular anterior scleritis. The appearance after removal of the scleral nodule from the right eye. Histology did not reveal a diagnostic cause.

Rheumatoid nodule of the sclera

5.19–5.22 Rheumatoid nodules of the sclera are uncommon. They rarely if ever require treatment and usually resolve spontaneously like this one. They should not be biopsied.

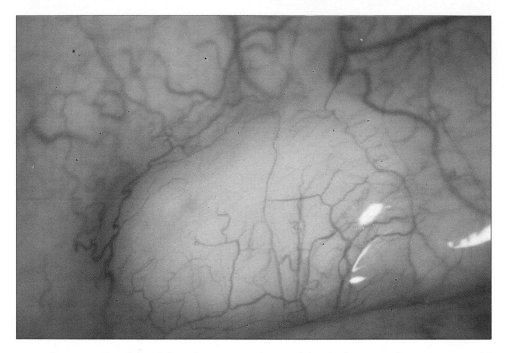

5.19 Rheumatoid nodule of the sclera. A painless nodule which occurred in a 59-year-old woman with long-standing articular rheumatoid arthritis. Two years later she developed vasculitic lesions on the legs and further nodules on the elbow.

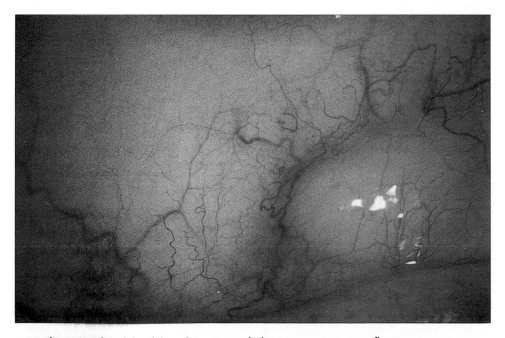

5.20 Rheumatoid nodule of the sclera. Arterial phase anterior segment fluorescein angiogram. There is diffuse leakage into the sclera initially and maximally at the site of the nodule. The vessels around the nodule are dilated but non-perfused. The black dots are spots of fluorescein.

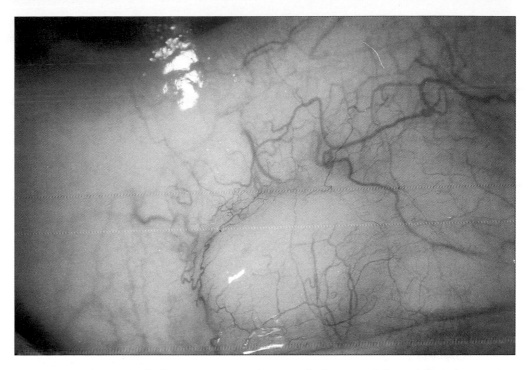

5.21 Venous phase. The leakage is now spreading outside the area of the nodule, indicating that the changes are not confined to the visible nodule.

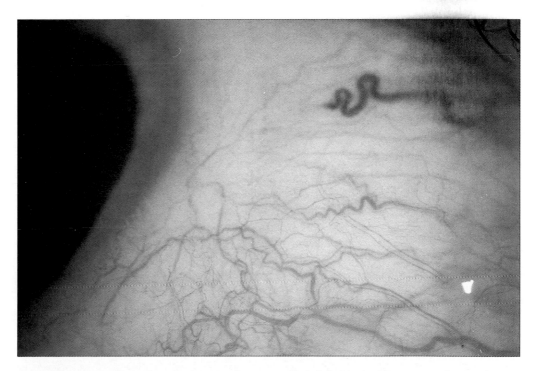

5.22 Late venous phase. The sclera is now almost completely full of leaked fluorescein. This is indicative of rheumatoid vasculitis, which needs to be treated systemically.

Necrotizing scleritis

Necrotizing scleritis is the most severe form of scleral disease and is almost always associated with some systemic disease. If misdiagnosed or left untreated, the patient will rapidly become blind, either because of perforation of the globe or the associated complications of keratitis, cataract or retinal oedema.

If uveitis is present it is certain that there is serious significant disease at or behind the equator of the globe.

Necrotizing scleritis with inflammation

The commonest form of necrotizing scleritis is accompanied by severe inflammation. The onset may be gradual, but inflammation often rises to a peak of intensity within a week of onset. It may be either unilateral or bilateral. The pain, which wakes the patient at night, occurs at the same time as the redness, but at this stage the physical signs may be minimal (**5.23, 5.24**) even though the patient is obviously ill. If the patient is inadequately treated, the sclera and overlying episclera and conjunctiva become necrotic within a very short time. This process will rapidly extend from the site of the original lesion, especially if the vascular tree is affected (**5.25–5.38**). However, intensive and adequate systemic therapy will reverse the situation and allow healing to occur. This healing is usually completed with fibrous tissue, but if the defect is too large the underlying choroid may be exposed (**5.39–5.49**).

In the early stages, low-dose anterior segment fluorescein angiography can be very helpful in deciding whether necrosis might occur. In necrotizing scleritis, as well as a deep leakage of dye, there are also vaso-occlusive changes in the overlying vessels and a gross abnormality of the adjacent limbal arcades (**5.50–5.55**). If these changes are seen, urgent systemic treatment is required.

Necrotizing scleritis without inflammation (scleromalacia perforans)

The term scleromalacia perforans should be used solely for patients who present with a necrosis of the sclera which is not accompanied by pain or severe ocular inflammation. Almost all patients with this condition have long-standing inactive rheumatoid arthritis. The changes in the sclera are almost always due to arteriolar occlusive changes, which result in death and sequestration of the affected tissue. As the changes are irreversible patients with this condition do not need treatment unless the disease is seen in its very early stages or there are other changes in the eye which need treating (**5.56–5.65**).

Anterior necrotizing scleritis

5.23–5.38 This 56-year-old white male patient presented with an intensely painful left eye with pain radiating to the head and jaw, which was waking him at night. The eye was tender above, but only slightly congested. The perforating vessels above were very dilated and there was some slight underlying scleral swelling (5.23). At 3 o'clock there was a corneal infiltrate and the limbal capillary nets were slightly distorted (5.24). Anterior segment fluorescein angiogram (5.25–5.27) revealed an extremely delayed perfusion of the vessels, the first dye appearing in the vessels 60 sec after injection (5.26). The patient returned a week later with an area of infarcted necrotic sclera in the area where the perforating vessels were seen to be dilated (5.28). These vessels appear to have been completely occluded and the adjacent tissue has become necrotic and infarcted. Tufts of new vessels can be seen to be entering the infarcted area. The vessels adjacent to the infarcted area fill early and completely but the larger vessels do not fill at all. The iris vessels in this segment are not affected.

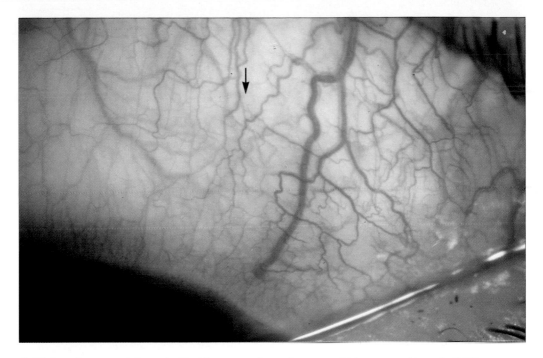

5.23 Anterior necrotizing scleritis. The arrow shows the area which necrosed later in **5.28**.

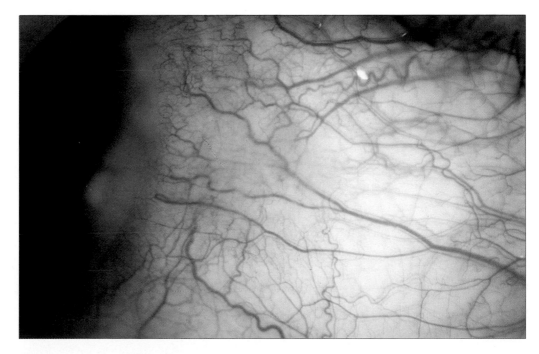

5.24 Anterior necrotizing scleritis.

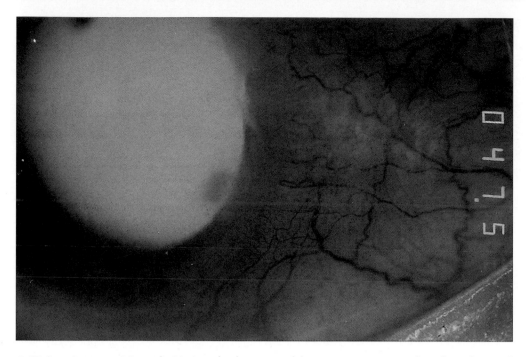

5.25 Anterior necrotizing scleritis. No dye has entered the eye at 47 sec even though perfusion of the other eye and the lid vessels was normal.

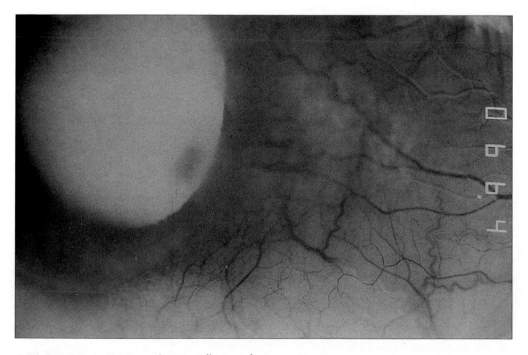

5.26 Anterior necrotizing scleritis. Still no perfusion at 66 sec.

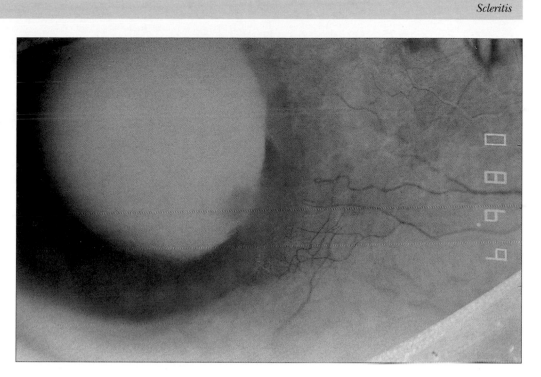

5.27 Anterior necrotizing scleritis. A very small amount of blood entering the circulation inferiorly at 86 sec.

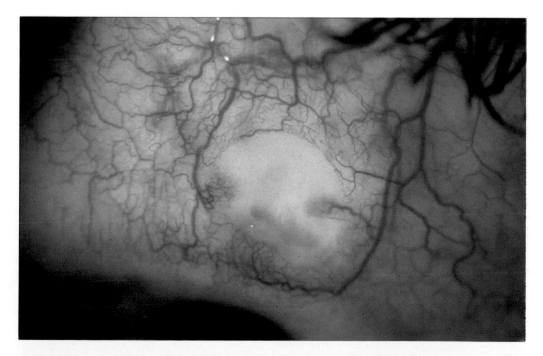

5.28 Anterior necrotizing scleritis. There was no indication in **5.23** that this necrotic area was likely to develop. Note how new vessels are entering the infarcted area only 24 hours after intensive therapy and how new vessels have spread around the limbus only one week after the start of ulceration.

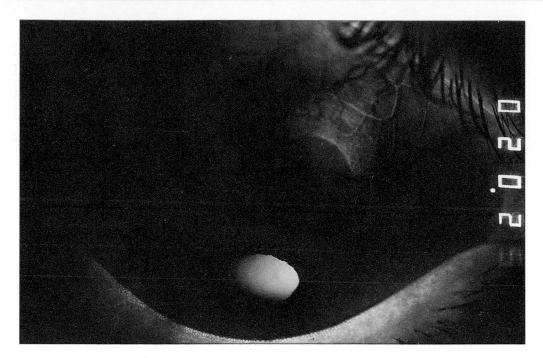

5.29 Anterior necrotizing scleritis. In response to the necrosis and consequent new vessel formation, the area adjacent to the necrotic spot is perfused but there is still no perfusion elsewhere in the anterior segment.

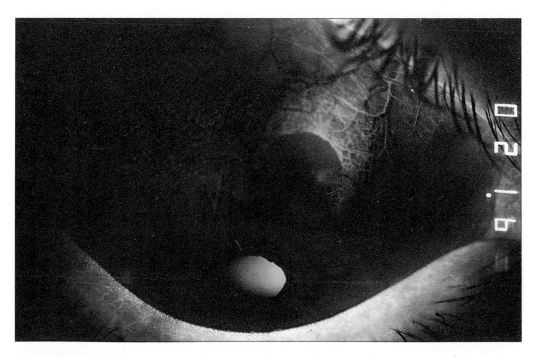

5.30 Anterior necrotizing scleritis. The new vessels seem to be arising from conjunctival vessels; note that the lid vessels are perfusing normally.

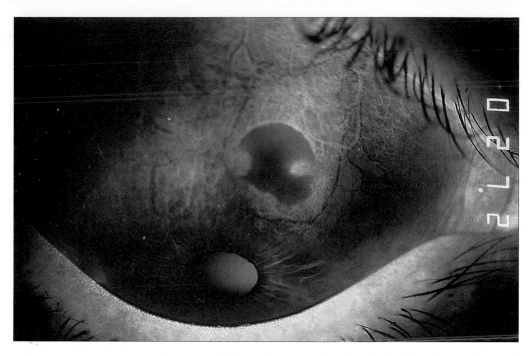

5.31 Anterior necrotizing scleritis. Rapid filling of new vessels in the depth of the ulcer. Perfusion of the limbus is limited but not in the region of the new large vessel.

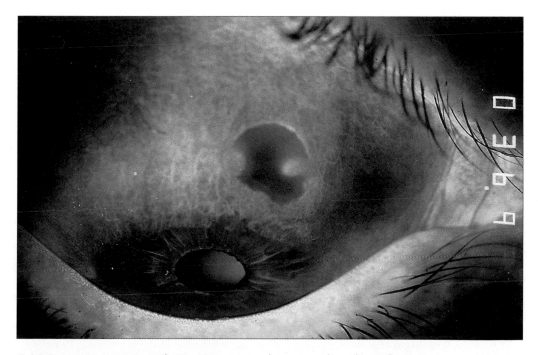

5.32 Anterior necrotizing scleritis. Late venous phase. Note how the perfusion remains in the area of the ulceration and that the limbal circulation has become permanently altered.

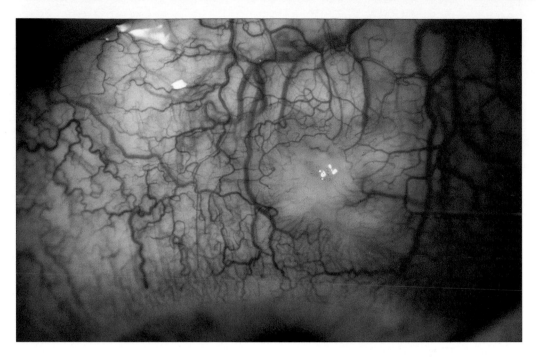

5.33 Anterior necrotizing scleritis. The lesion healed with treatment, but the patient had recurrent attacks of scleritis.

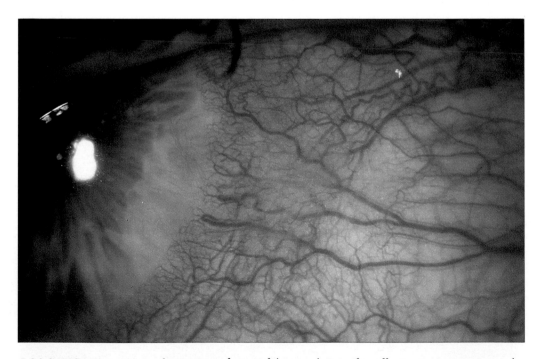

5.34 Anterior necrotizing scleritis. Reperfusion of the circulation after effective treatment 12 months later. Note how the limbal infiltrates seen in **5.24** have disappeared and in this area the superficial limbal arcades are normal even though the episcleral arteries have become multiple and dilated.

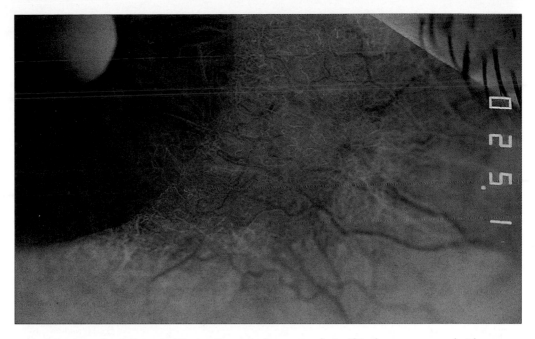

5.35 Anterior necrotizing scleritis. Angiogram taken a year later. This shows new vessels. The superficial new vessels which had grown into the cornea are looped (indicating a lack of activity) at the site where there had previously been poor perfusion and corneal infiltration. The long straight vessels which were derived from the deep episcleral plexus are deep within corneal tissue. There is no leakage from the tips (they are therefore inactive) but they are unable to loop up with neighbouring vessels because of the tight collagen structure of the cornea.

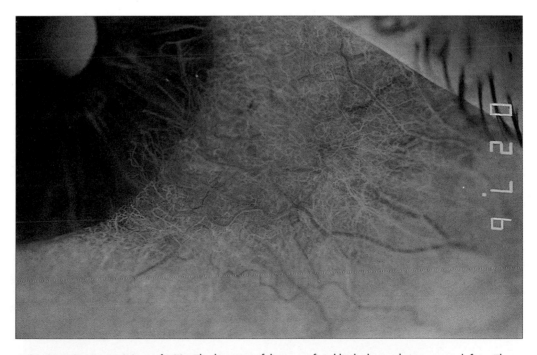

5.36 Anterior necrotizing scleritis. The looping of the superficial limbal vessels is easy to define. These vessels do not leak. Note however that the adjacent limbus is still hypoperfused.

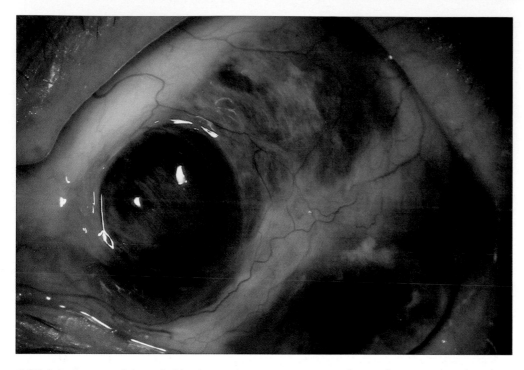

5.37 Anterior necrotizing scleritis. Severe anterior necrotizing scleritis after treatment. The sclera remains thin in the area of active disease and is complete in another. The limbal circulation is compromised, leading to some peripheral corneal change. No treatment is required at this stage, as the eye is not threatened by the absence of scleral tissue.

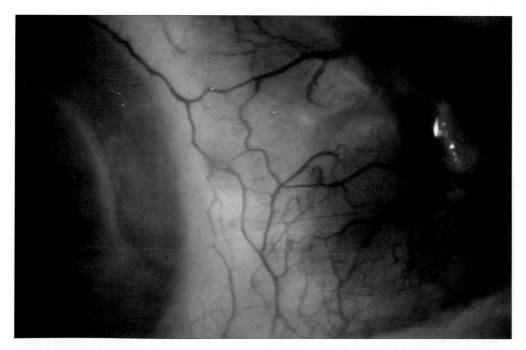

5.38 Anterior necrotizing scleritis. The hypoperfused zone at the limbus has contributed to the loss of tissue in the cornea which is also involved in the necrosis caused by the intense inflammatory response.

Anterior necrotizing scleritis

5.39–5.49 *Severe necrotizing sclerokeratitis in a 61-year-old man at presentation (**5.39–5.41**). There are numerous avascular necrotic areas in the sclera, and the cornea is infiltrated, oedematous and vascularized from the limbus.*

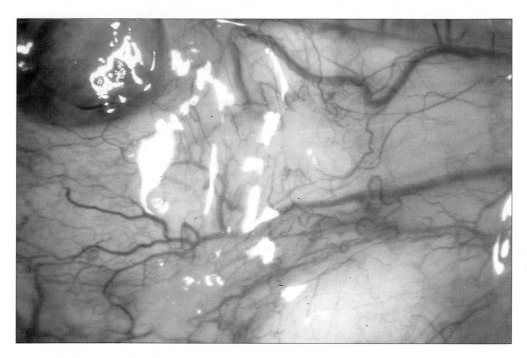

5.39 Multiple hypoperfused areas adjacent to an area of total tissue loss. These avascular areas are over an area of active scleral necrosis.

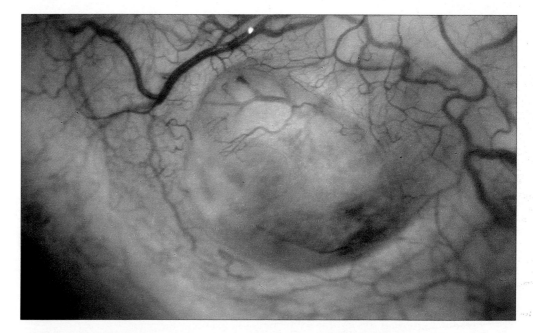

5.40 Anterior necrotizing scleritis. Loss of scleral tissue together with the overlying episclera and part of the conjunctiva.

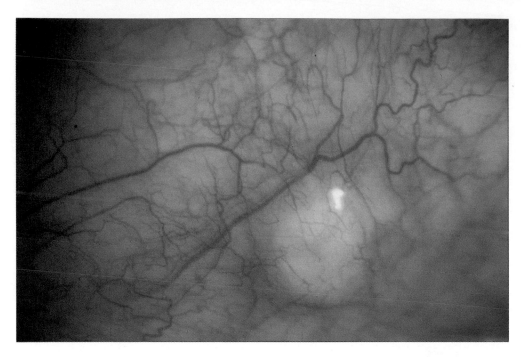

5.41 Anterior necrotizing scleritis. An area of necrotizing sclera and hypoperfused conjunctiva and episclera, at presentation.

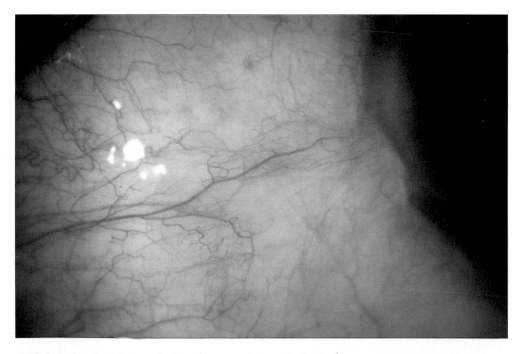

5.42 Anterior necrotizing scleritis. The same area as in **5.41** after treatment.

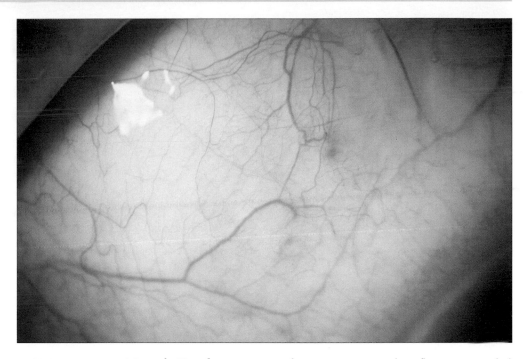

5.43 Anterior necrotizing scleritis. After one course of systemic treatment the inflammation settled without further recurrence. Five years later the large necrotic area had only a very thin conjunctival cover but the choroid only bulged slightly and there was no inflammation. Elsewhere, the necrotic tissue had been replaced by apparently normal tissue and the cornea was clear (**5.45–5.49**).

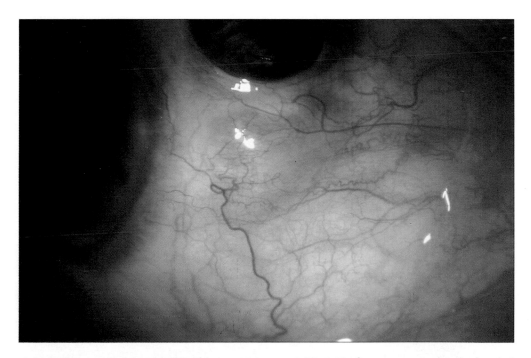

5.44 Anterior necrotizing scleritis. The same area as in **5.39, 5.40** after treatment with pulsed methyl prednisolone and cyclophosphamide.

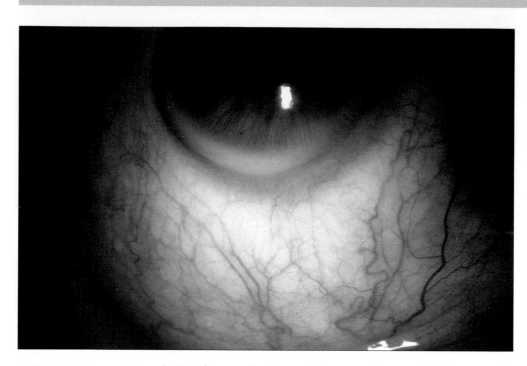

5.45 Anterior necrotizing scleritis. This area had three early necrotic lesions which disappeared within 24 hours of starting therapy.

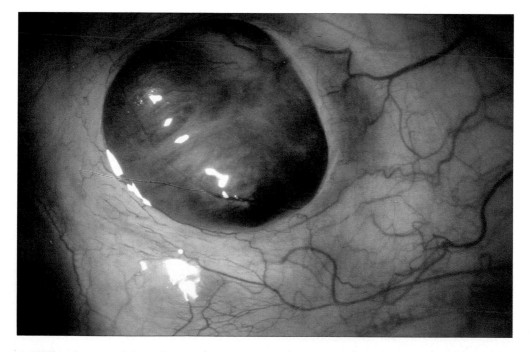

5.46 Anterior necrotizing scleritis. The appearance three years after treatment. There have been no further recurrences after a four-month treatment course at the end of which all treatment with steroids and cyclophosphamide was withdrawn.

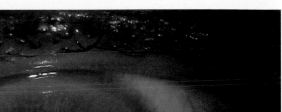

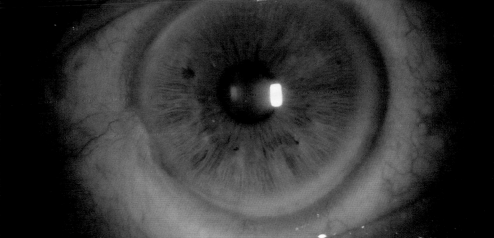

5.47 Anterior necrotizing scleritis. Appearance after treatment.

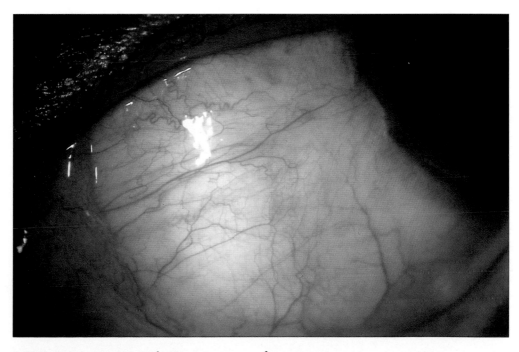

5.48 Anterior necrotizing scleritis. Appearance after treatment.

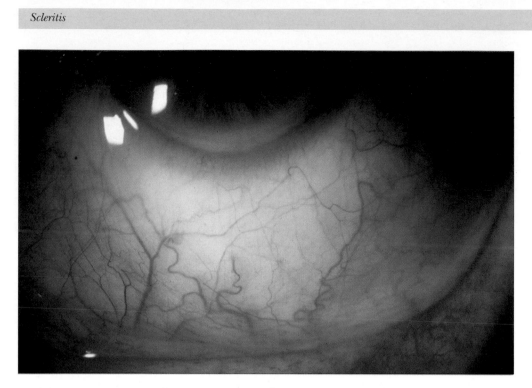

5.49 Anterior necrotizing scleritis. Appearance after treatment.

Early anterior necrotizing scleritis

5.50–5.55 This 57-year-old man with severe rheumatoid arthritis presented with an active anterior scleritis. Fluorescein angiography revealed early deep scleral leakage of dye, a totally occluded episcleral vessel, disruption of the limbal arcades with budding of new vessels and leakage of dye into the cornea.

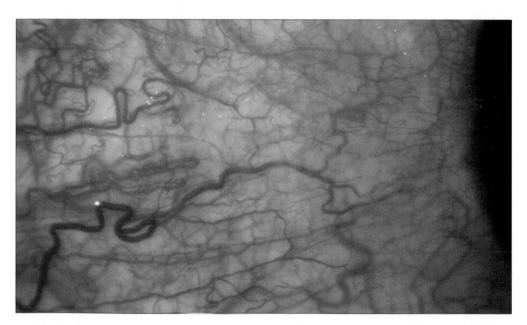

5.50 Early anterior necrotizing scleritis. The appearance at presentation. The eye does not appear to have any serious inflammation although there is obvious congestion of vessels in the limbal area and some destruction of the vascular patterns.

5.51 Early anterior necrotizing scleritis. Early arterial phase. There is immediate deep leakage into the perilimbal areas and an obvious abnormality of the vascular networks.

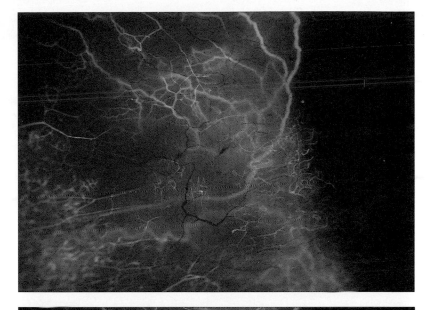

5.52 Early anterior necrotizing scleritis. Late arterial phase. all the vessels filling here are new vessels – mostly derived from conjunctiva. They leak and almost all terminate in blind endings.

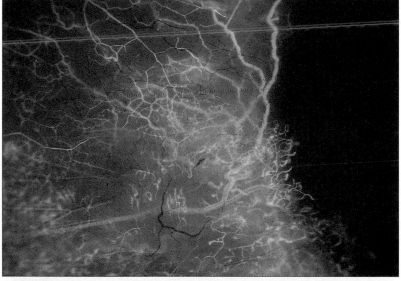

5.53 Early anterior necrotizing scleritis. Early venous phase. A similar pattern showing the same limbal arcade changes. Histologically this pattern indicates migration of lymphocytes into an area of inflammation.

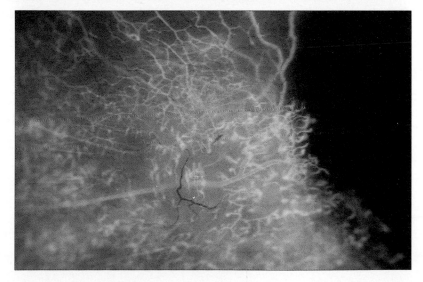

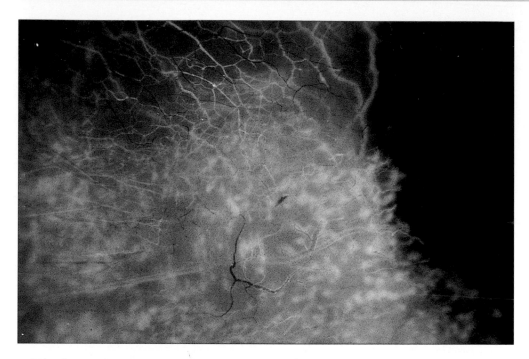

5.54 Early anterior necrotizing scleritis. Late venous phase.

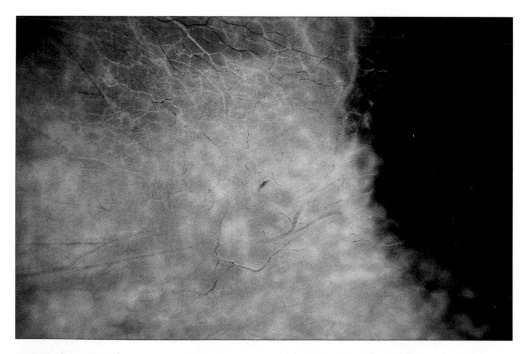

5.55 Early anterior necrotizing scleritis. Late venous phase. The leakage has become widespread involving vessels not apparently affected in the early phases of the angiography.

Necrotizing scleritis without inflammation

5.56–5.65 *This 78-year-old woman had had rheumatoid arthritis for many years. She had severe crippling deformity of the hands, knees and elbows and was confined to a wheelchair, however, the rheumatoid arthritis was no longer active. She presented with a feeling of slight discomfort and an 'unusual appearance' of the sclera.*

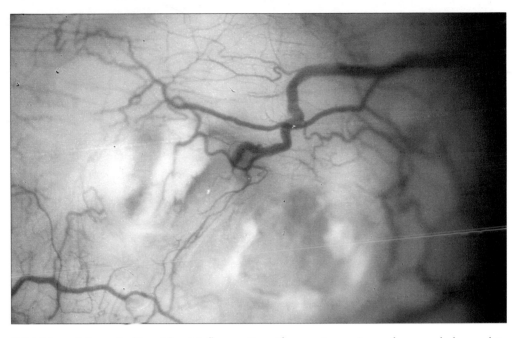

5.56 Necrotizing scleritis without inflammation. Fluorescein angiography revealed complete capillary non-perfusion over this area. At presentation, even though the conjunctiva, episclera and sclera are actively thinning, there is little surrounding inflammation.

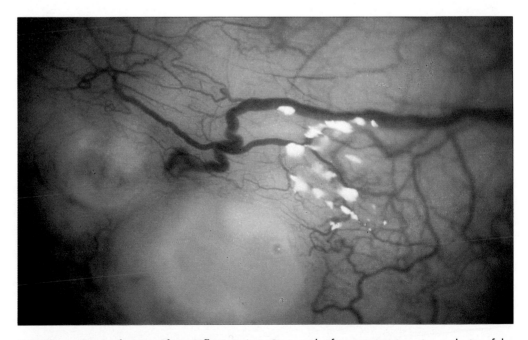

5.57 Necrotizing scleritis without inflammation. One week after presentation. Avascularity of the conjunctiva and episclera in an area adjacent to **5.56.**

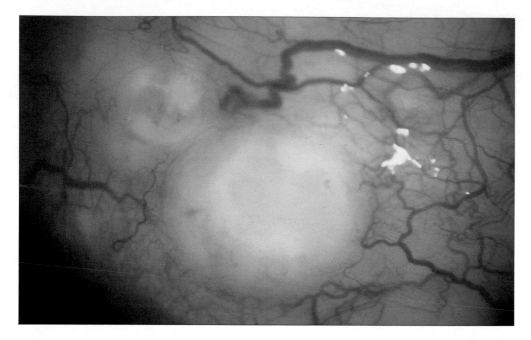

5.58 Necrotizing scleritis without inflammation. The area seen in **5.56** two weeks after presentation. The area of ischemia is larger and now incorporates a smaller similar lesion next to it.

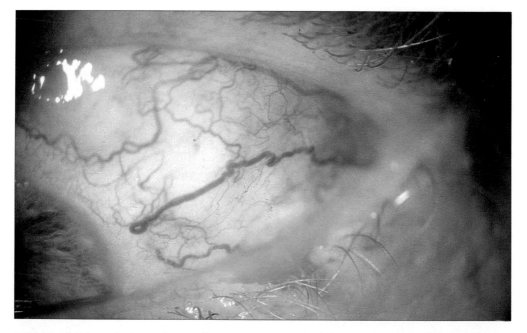

5.59 Necrotizing scleritis without inflammation. One month later. At this stage the necrotic area does not stain.

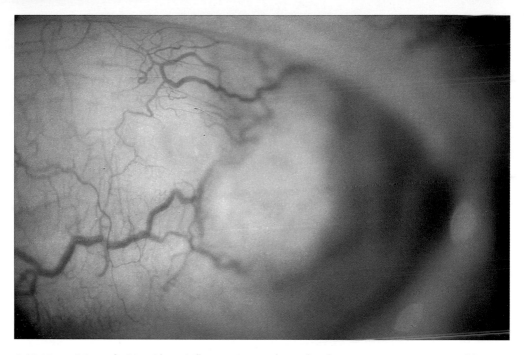

5.60 Necrotizing scleritis without inflammation. Eight weeks after presentation. Staining of the two areas seen in **5.58** as the conjunctiva also becomes necrotic.

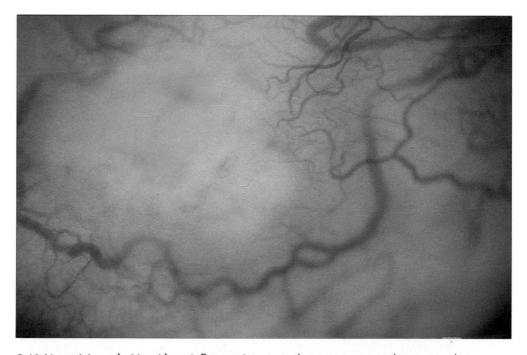

5.61 Necrotizing scleritis without inflammation. A similar appearance in the superior lesion of **5.59**.

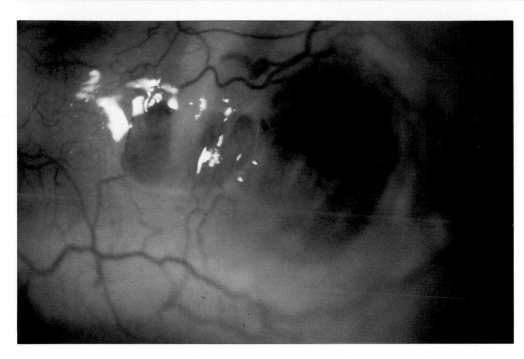

5.62 Necrotizing scleritis without inflammation. Twelve months later this and all the surrounding area of sclera had become resorbed.

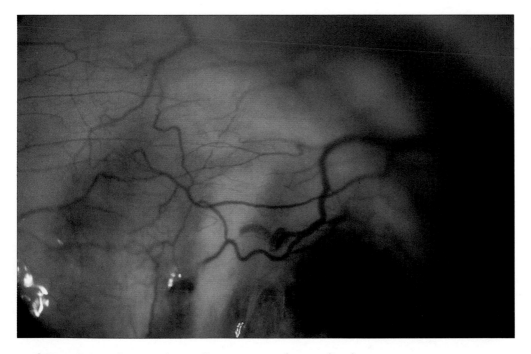

5.63 Necrotizing scleritis without inflammation. Twelve months after presentation.

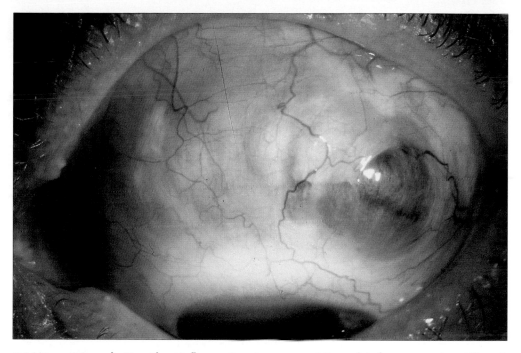

5.64 Necrotizing scleritis without inflammation. Appearance 18 months after presentation. Although most of the sclera in the affected area has been resorbed, there is only a small staphyloma in one area.

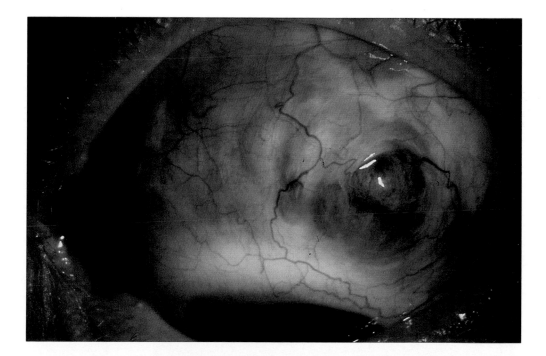

5.65 Necrotizing scleritis without inflammation. Appearance three years after presentation. Staphylomas do not occur provided the intraocular pressure remains normal. Any glaucoma in a scleritis patient needs to be controlled by: firstly, controlling the inflammation, and secondly, treating with anti-glaucoma medication. If surgery has to be performed this must be done in an area where there is the most normal conjunctiva and sclera.

Posterior sceritis

Posterior sceritis is very under-diagnosed. It is not uncommon, but it presents in such a variety of ways that it is often not considered in the differential diagnosis of visual loss, particularly if pain is not a prominent feature.

There appear to be two major sub-groupings of posterior sceritis:

- In young people who complain of rapidly decreasing visual acuity and a variable amount of pain which is often referred outside the eye. The commonest physical sign is of choroidal folds and/or swelling of the optic nerve head. No anterior sceritis or systemic disease can be found (**5.66, 5.67**).
- Other patients present in a similar way to those who have anterior sceritis. In some instances the disease spreads from the anterior segment; in others it starts in the posterior segment and can be diffuse (**5.66–5.68**), nodular (**5.69, 5.70**) or necrotizing (**5.71**). As in anterior sceritis, many patients have associated systemic disease (**5.72–5.80**).

Posterior sceritis has become much more frequently recognized since the advent of the 90D lens, fluorescein angiography, B-scan ultrasonography and CT scanning. Also ophthalmologists have become much more aware of the possibility of posterior sceritis being the cause in unusual cases of loss of vision, exudative detachments, choroidal effusion syndrome, swollen discs and choroidal folds.

B-scan ultrasonography is by far the most useful investigation in this condition. The features which need to be looked for on ultrasonography are:

- The thickness of the posterior coats of the eye beyond the normal range of 1.2–1.9 mm. It is not possible to distinguish retina, sclera and choroid from each other unless they are detached.
- Separation of the posterior surface of the sclera from the episclera.
- Presence or absence of retinal or choroidal detachments, or swelling of the disc (**5.81**).

If ultrasonography is not available, CT scanning can give useful information. MRI scanning does not seem to give much more information than ultrasonography or CT scanning.

Posterior sceritis

5.66–5.68 A 45-year-old white male presented with reduction of vision and some pain in the left eye. He was found to have shallowing of the anterior chamber and raised intraocular pressure; swelling of the posterior coats of the eye to 3.2 mm (normal 1.2–1.9 mm); and unusual but marked choroidal folds which crossed the macula. No systemic disease was found and the condition resolved in this instance without treatment.

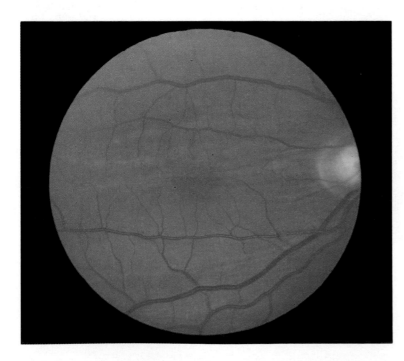

5.66 Posterior sceritis. Fundus appearance of choroidal folds.

5.67 Posterior scleritis. Post-segment fluorescein angiogram. Choroidal folds cross the macula in the same patient as **5.66** in the region of the swelling seen in **5.68**.

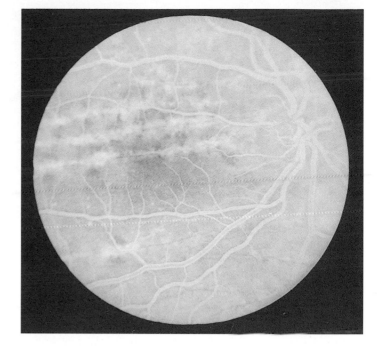

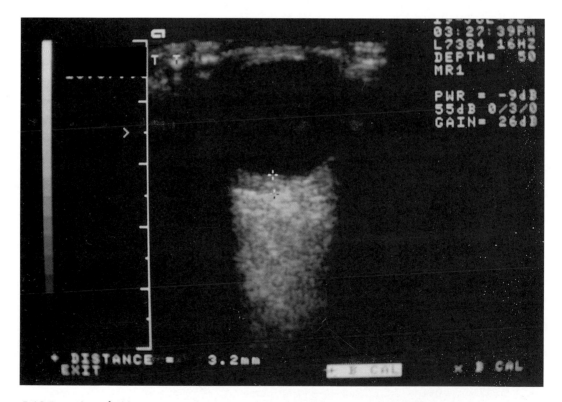

5.68 Posterior scleritis.

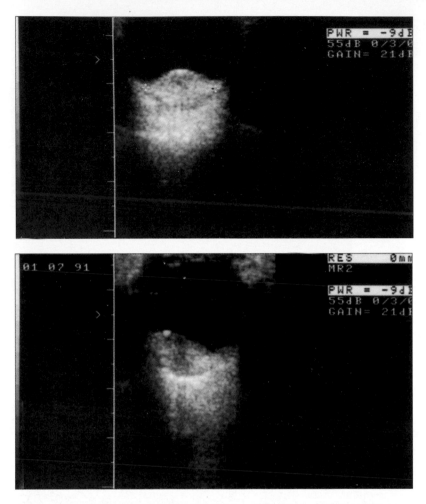

5.69, 5.70 Nodular posterior scleritis. A large nodule presenting in a 35-year-old male with no systemic disease. He had minimal choroidal folds but multiple pigment epithelial defects on angiography.

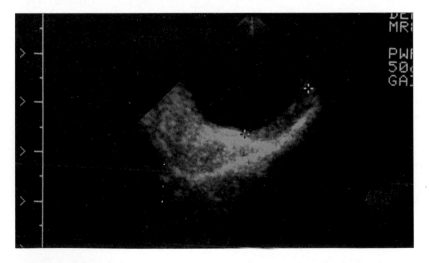

5.71 Necrotizing posterior scleritis. This unusual appearance of a thick, extensive destructive lesion of the posterior sclera occurred in a 59-year-old patient with periarteritis nodosa.

Posterior scleritis

5.72–5.80 *This 24-year-old white female had developed a 'full' feeling on the left side of her face at the age of 18 and had had difficulty moving her eyes from side to side. She had been admitted to hospital with a diagnosis of possible meningitis and the condition resolved without treatment. Three years later she had a similar episode with purulent discharge from the left nostril and poor vision with a central scotoma in the left eye. This cleared rapidly with systemic steroid. She again remained symptom-free for three years when she again presented with poor vision, pain in the face and this time a weak voice. Examination showed macula oedema. ANCA (Anti-nuclear cytoplasmic antibodies) were positive so she was treated with steroids and cyclosporin. An ultrasound scan 5 months later shows an almost normal sclera. Her current therapy is cyclosporin and 5 mg prednisolone on alternate days. Her symptoms, nasal biopsy and a positive cANCA confirmed the diagnosis of Wegener's granulomatosis.* (Courtesy of Mr Paul, Wolverhampton.)

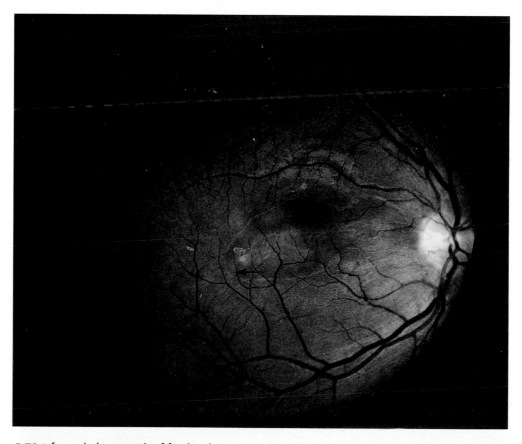

5.72 Infra-red photograph of fundus showing marked retinal oedema caused by a localized area of choroidal/scleral swelling.

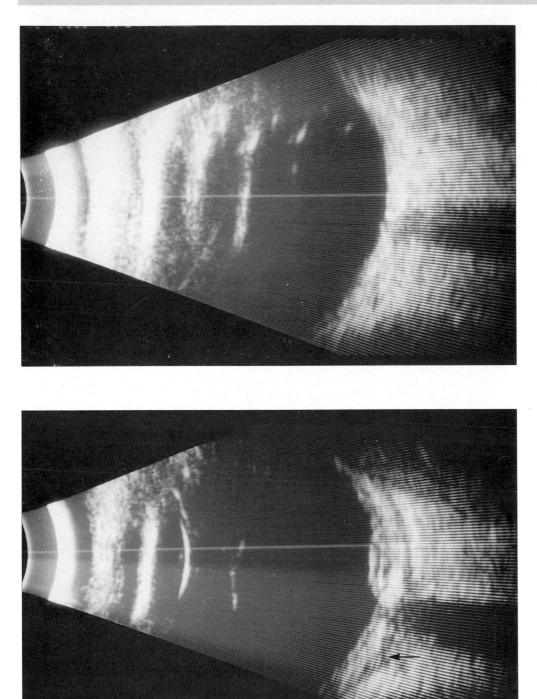

5.73, 5.74 Posterior scleritis. Right eye (**5.73**) and left eye (**5.74**). B-scan ultrasound shows a thickened posterior sclera with separation of the episcleral space, indicating oedema of the ocular coats (arrowed) and an overlying macular oedema.

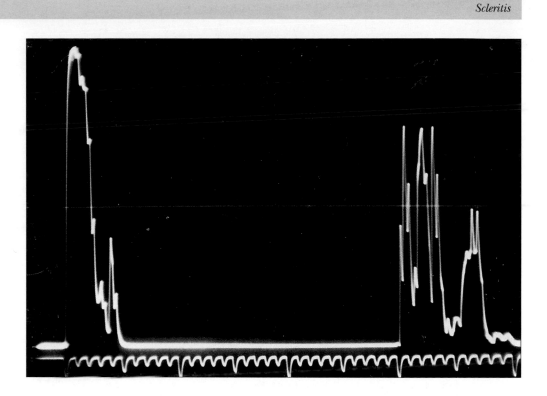

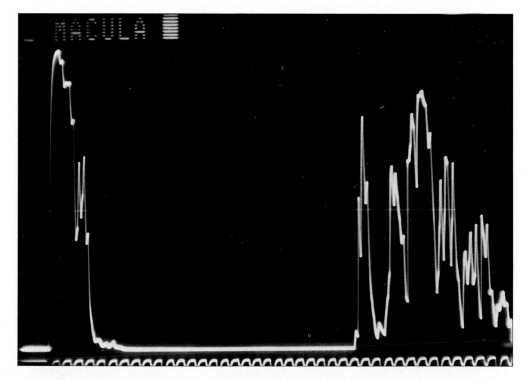

5.75, 5.76 Posterior scleritis. Right eye (**5.75**) and left eye (**5.76**). A-scans of same patient as in **5.73, 5.74** before treatment.

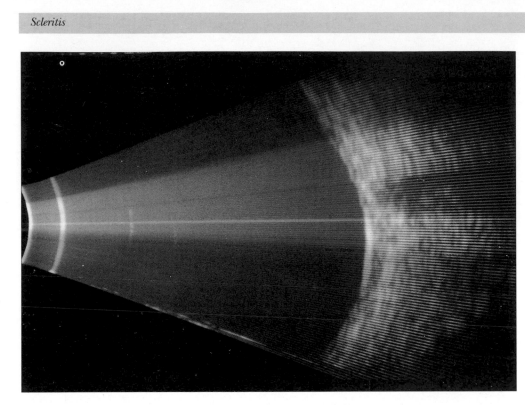

5.77 Posterior scleritis. Right eye. B-scan of same patient as in **5.72–5.76** after treatment. Although there is still some slight infiltrate around the optic nerve, the sclera is of normal thickness.

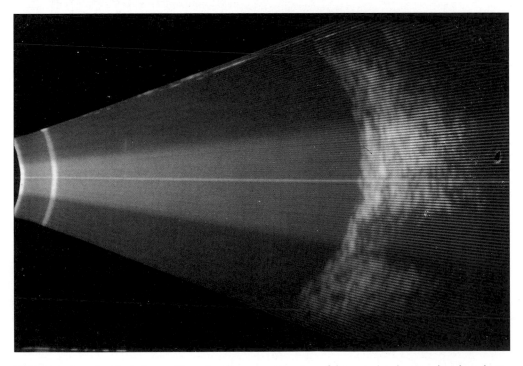

5.78 Posterior scleritis. Left eye. There is still some separation of the episcleral space, but the scleritis is now of normal thickness and there is no macular oedema.

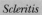

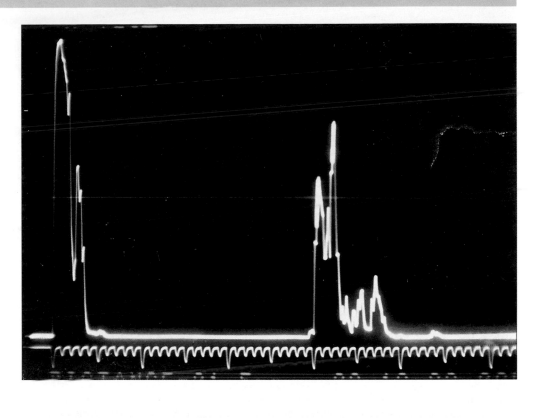

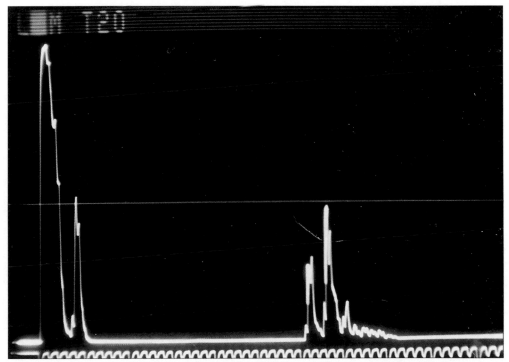

5.79, 5.80 Posterior scleritis. Right eye (**5.79**) and left eye (**5.80**). A-scans in same patient as **5.75, 5.76** and at the same settings, showing the reduction of echoes following treatment.

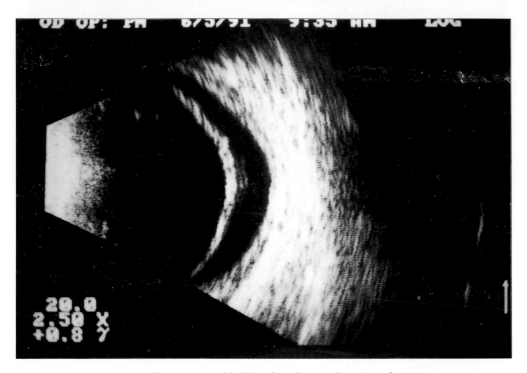

5.81 Posterior scleritis. This 65-year-old white female was known to have severe Wegener's granulomatosis and had had severe anterior necrotizing scleritis which had come under control with treatment. She had been well for a year when, within 24 hours, her vision faded and she developed a choroidal effusion with some thickening of the sclera. She rapidly responded to further systemic treatment.

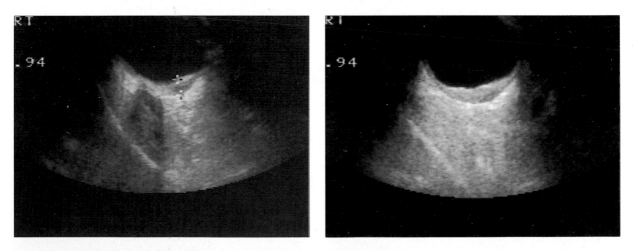

5.82, 5.83 Posterior scleritis. A 53-year-old woman who complained of intermittant severe pain accompanied by diminution of vision. The vision returned and the pain has been relieved by steroid cyclophosphamide treatment. The patient requires 7.5 mg prednisolone and 50 mg cyclophosphamide daily to keep her symptom free.

The management of scleritis

Unlike episcleritis, scleritis is a potentially destructive disease. Patients with this condition must always be thoroughly investigated as most will have some underlying systemic, vascular or connective tissue disorder. The underlying systemic disorder must be treated and this may in itself be sufficient to control the ocular disease. However, because of the unusual immunological situation in the eye, adjunctive therapy is almost always required.

Local steroid therapy is of no value in scleral disease. It may improve the patient's comfort, but it has no effect in suppressing the inflammation.

Scleritis is largely associated with the seropositive connective tissue disorders, and is immunologically induced and perpetuated. It is also often associated with a systemic autoimmune vasculitis. These disorders must be specifically looked for and excluded.

Anterior diffuse and nodular scleritis, although found in patients with connective tissue disorders, are rarely sight-threatening and often respond to non-steroidal anti-inflammatory drugs (NSAIDs). However, necrotizing scleritis is rapidly destructive and requires urgent treatment with immunosuppressive therapy. Posterior scleritis is more difficult to manage because of the difficulties in the differential diagnosis, but the same principles apply and control of pain is by far the best indicator of success of treatment.

Therapeutic regimes for scleral disease

Patients with diffuse, nodular anterior scleritis and their counterparts in the posterior segment will usually respond to an NSAID. Not all of those on the market are equally effective. Our current practice is to use flurbiprofen 100 mg three times a day until the disease is suppressed.

As soon as the eye is quiet, the drug may be withdrawn as it is unusual for the disease to recur immediately. Some patients may develop side effects. The gastric side effects are usually treatable with ranitidine or equivalent drugs but sometimes the NSAID has to be withdrawn completely. Change to another preparation is rarely successful.

Control can be reliably measured by the presence or absence of pain and by the degree of swelling and vascular congestion. The presence or absence of pain may also be used to titrate the dosage of medication; for example the initial dosage required to control the inflammatory response in one patient was 100 mg flurbiprofen three times a day. The treatment was stopped after 10 days but the pain and some inflammation recurred. He was pain free on a dosage of 50 mg morning and evening and 100 mg at midday, and had to remain on this dose for 3 months before treatment could eventually be withdrawn. Failure to control diffuse or nodular scleritis with an NSAID should make one suspect the presence of an early necrotizing scleritis. Also, if fluorescein angiography reveals an area of non-perfusion, this patient must be considered to have early necrotizing scleritis. If there is no immediate response to NSAIDs, the patient must be treated with immunosuppressants.

In patients with intractable disease, and those with necrotizing scleritis, systemic steroids should be given. These must be given in immunosuppressive dosages in order to control the disease, i.e. oral prednisolone 60–80 mg daily. As soon as the disease is under control (i.e. when the pain goes), the dose can rapidly be reduced to an anti-inflammatory dose of 20 mg, within 4 to 6 days, and then gradually withdrawn.

There are a few patients who will require additional therapy because the disease recurs when the steroids are reduced below 20 mg prednisolone. These patients require additional non-steroidal medication, so that the steroid requirement can be reduced. The combination therapy will often reduce the steroid requirement to 5 mg prednisolone or less. If this fails, cyclosporin should be considered. Azathioprine is often advocated as a steroid-sparing agent as well as an immunosuppressive agent. Unfortunately, this is not very effective in the treatment of scleritis. In patients with a systemic vasculitis, systemic cyclophosphamide will have to be given, the maintenance dosage being related to the lymphocyte count. There is always a delay in the therapeutic effect of this type of immunosuppressive agent. During this period, which lasts 2–3 weeks, high steroid dosage will have to be continued. In a further few cases, the disease is so severe and the eye so much at risk that pulsed therapy with intravenous prednisolone and cyclophosphamide should be considered. These regimes are potentially hazardous, and treatment should be undertaken with a physician or rheumatologist conversant with their use.

Surgery in necrotizing keratitis

Surgery should only be undertaken when the systemic disease has been brought under control, and continued supervision of both the eye and the systemic disease must be continued if the graft is to survive. Surgery may be required if the eye becomes perforated. The disease cannot be controlled when there is excess antigen load or if the patient is unable to take medication. Systemic intravenous pulsed steroid and immunosuppression must be given at the time of surgery. Lamellar grafting is ideal. The patient in Figures **5.84–5.87** was treated in this way and then given a double crescent-shaped graft which was completely incorporated into host tissue 6 years later (**5.87**).

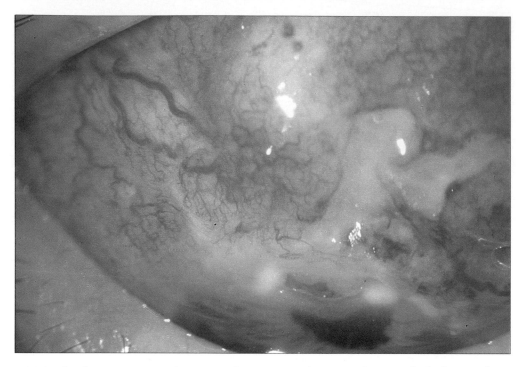

5.84 Localized Wegener's granulomatosis. There is severe destructive change at the limbus, involving both cornea and sclera. This is the most commonly presenting feature in this disease.

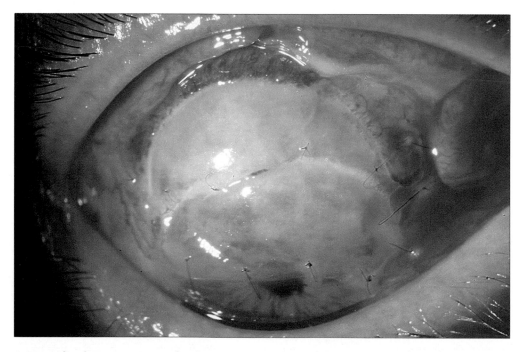

5.85 Localized Wegener's granulomatosis. Same patient as **5.84**. Treatment with intravenous methyl prednisolone 500 mg and pulsed cyclophosphamide 500 mg was given, but the globe perforated a few hours later. The perforation was sealed with cyanacrylate glue and a contact bandage lens. When the systemic disease had come under control a double lamellar graft was performed as the original perforation remained plugged with iris and there was no further leakage.

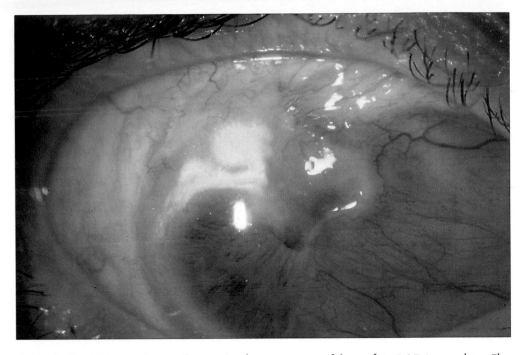

5.86 Localized Wegener's granulomatosis. The appearance of the graft in **5.85** 6 years later. The graft has become completely incorporated into the host tissue, even though it has largely opacified. There is a pseudopterygium inferonasally.

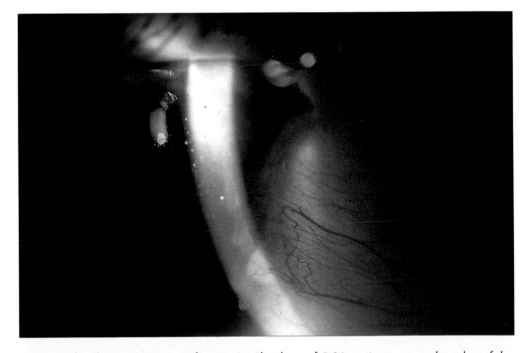

5.87 Localized Wegener's granulomatosis. Slit photo of **5.86** at six years, at the edge of the pseudopterygium. The cornea in this region is thinned and there are old keratic precipitates on the host cornea.

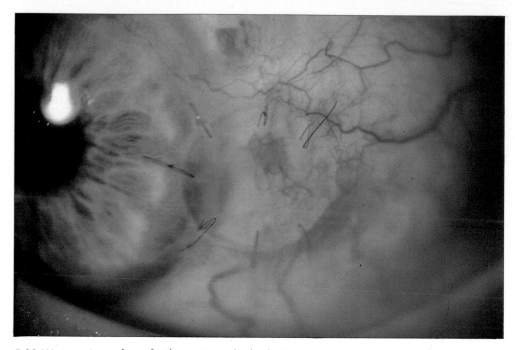

5.88 Wegener's patch graft. This patient who had Wegener's granulomatosis was well controlled with systemic steroids and cyclophosphamide except for one area on the limbus at 3 o'clock. The pain persisted at the site and the limbus became very thin. A small patch graft was successful in stopping the pain.

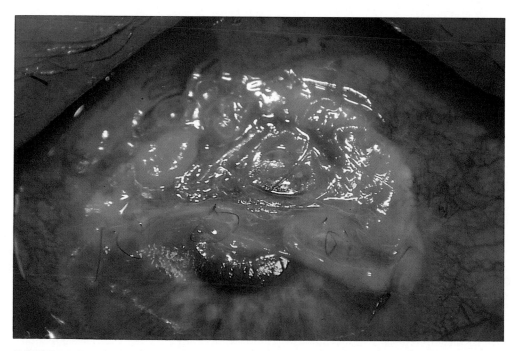

5.89 Necrosis recurring in a graft in an eye which had been treated with a lamellar keratoplasty for necrotizing scleritis. The graft was replaced and has remained clear.

6.
Corneal Involvement in Scleral Disease

The cornea may become involved at any stage during the course of episcleral or scleral inflammatory disease. The corneal changes are more commonly seen when the inflammation is severe and they are always preceded by easily identifiable changes to the limbal vasculature in which the vessels leak, become occluded or sprout new vessel complexes (**6.1–6.4**). As these changes are characteristic of the various conditions, careful observations of these vessels in the early stages of the scleral inflammation may give a clue as to the probable severity and possible progression of the disease. If there is excessive leakage, particularly from new vessels, this will lead to corneal opacification. It will also lead to lipid deposition and corneal infiltration as it interferes with the normal flow of metabolites within the corneal tissue. If on the other hand there are vasculitic changes within the limbal vessels, then changes occur within the circulation which may become totally or partially occluded as well as incompetant. These changes if prolonged lead to the formation of new vessels around the limbus and if there is an appropriate stimulus they will invade the cornea itself. Any of the vascular networks at the limbus, whether deep or superficial, can give rise to these new vessels (**6.4**). Inflammation adjacent to the limbus always disrupts the normal limbal architecture and cytokines are also released into the cornea as well as cells. The cytokines penetrate the cornea, widely affecting the corneal fibrocytes. If their concentration is very high, as in necrotizing scleritis, then the corneal tissue becomes damaged and resorbed leading to various and often characteristic peripheral and central corneal changes.

Corneal infiltration to the extent of opacification is most commonly seen in patients who have had scleritis following an attack of herpes zoster, and peripheral corneal tissue is most often lost as a result of a granuloma or vasculitis affecting the limbus. The limbal vasculitis and vascular occlusion may lead either to the gradual loss of the peripheral corneal tissue or an active destruction of tissue. Gradual corneal loss is epitomized by the 'contact lens cornea' in which the central cornea remains normal whilst the periphery becomes extremely thin (**6.11, 6.12**). This contrasts with the changes seen in the more severe inflammatory problems in which the tissue destruction can be so rapid that ulceration of the overlying epithelium occurs (**6.14**). Thus several types of corneal changes associated with scleritis can be identified. In the diffuse and nodular forms the cornea becomes infiltrated and sometimes vascularized in regions adjacent to the inflamed sclera (**6.7**). These changes are much more likely to occur if the attacks are recurrent, severe or poorly treated. Ulceration and deep guttering do not occur in this situation. In necrotizing disease the changes are more intense. Some are related only to the adjacent necrotizing scleritis (**6.13**). In this situation, the cornea becomes damaged as a result of the cellular and cytokine activity associated with the original disease. Other patients may develop localized or circumferential corneal changes (**6.9**). The destructive change once initiated in the cornea can sometimes progress separately from the scleral disease and can become so severe that perforation can result (**7.5, 8.3**). Finally, the cornea can be invaded by a granuloma arising in the episcleral tissue. Such a granuloma destroys both the sclera and cornea around it by degrading the collagenous tissue (**6.20–6.22**).

The patients shown in **6.5** and **6.15–6.17** all developed sclerokeratitis of different types following an attack of herpes zoster ophthalmicus. Their responses were all different because the sclerokeratitis was not caused directly by the virus but by the immune response to the virus and the tissue reactions resulting from the immune response. Scleral disease results from a combination of a trigger factor (often an infective organism), the site of the initial infection or initiating stimulus, the type and intensity of the immune response to the stimulus, and the genetic make-up of the individual. Thus the same sequence of responses can occur following a bacterial infection or following simple surgical trauma (SINS), if the patient is appropriately sensitized at the time when the insult occurs (see Chapter 8).

Corneal changes in scleral disease

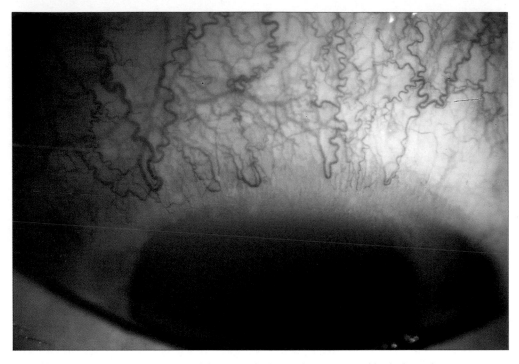

6.1 Systemic vasculitis. A 57-year-old man with the earliest stages of limbal involvement. Note the grey infiltrates at the tips of the limbal vascular arcades. The cornea in this region is infiltrated, but there has been no vascular remodelling or new vessel formation so far.

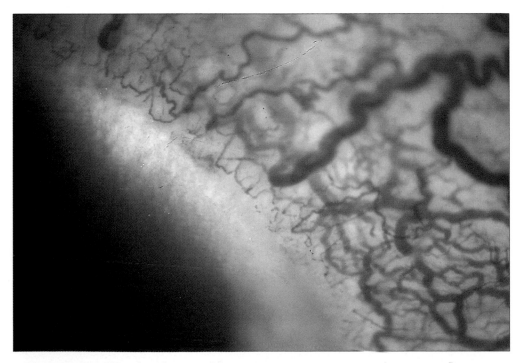

6.2 Systemic vasculitis. The other eye of the same patient as in **6.1**. Note the intense inflammation of the sclera and episclera, however, the blood is static in the limbal arcades. There are some fine haemorrhages and the cornea has become infiltrated.

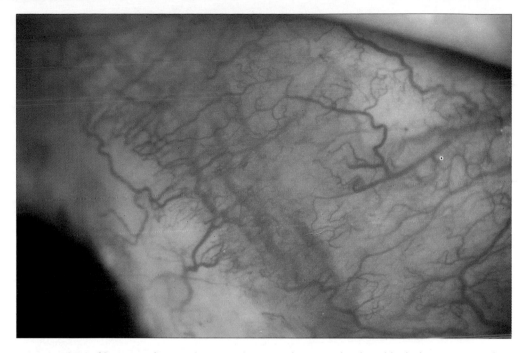

6.3 Vascular infiltration of an early corneal gutter. There is scleral and limbal congestion. The limbal arcades are disrupted and new vessels pass to the centrally advancing edge. The leading edge of the vessels leaks.

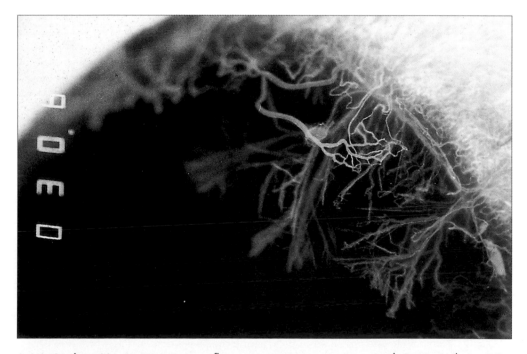

6.4 Active keratitis. Anterior segment fluorescein angiogram in an active keratitis similar to **6.3**. New vessels arise both from the superficial limbal arcades and from the deeper vessels of the long posterior ciliary vessels. Both sets are straight and invade the stroma. Each vessel is separate from its origin and not looped to its fellow. This indicates activity of the keratitis.

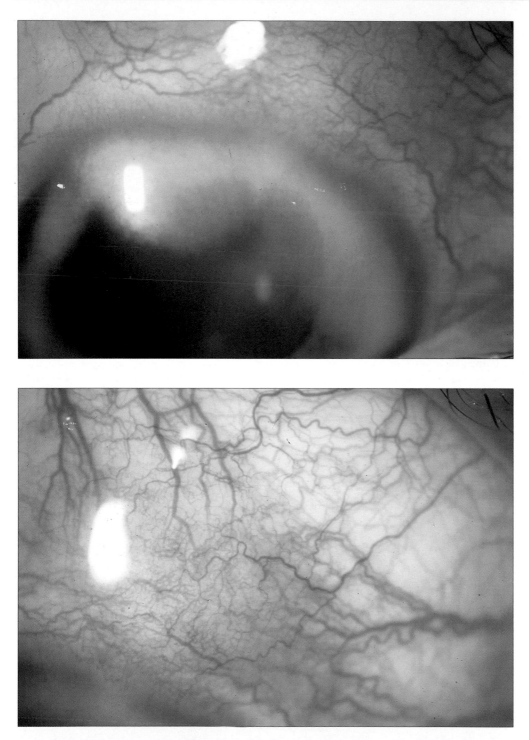

6.5, 6.6 Following herpes zoster ophthalmicus this 70-year-old Pakistani woman developed a severe diffuse anterior scleritis 6 weeks after the start of the disease. The scleritis persisted and the cornea gradually became infiltrated with lipid as a result of incompetent new vessels which had arisen from the limbal arcades.

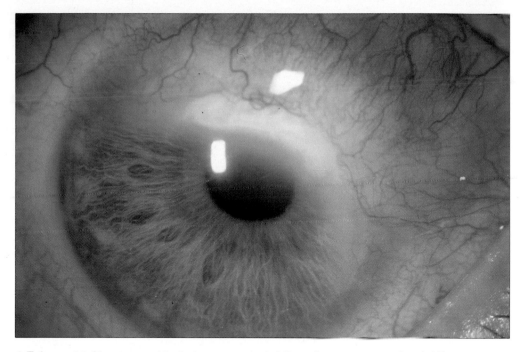

6.7 Corneal infiltration and limbal pannus which followed numerous attacks of diffuse anterior scleritis in the upper sclera. Once new incompetent vessels had infiltrated the peripheral corneal tissue, the condition progressed in spite of adequate control of the scleritis.

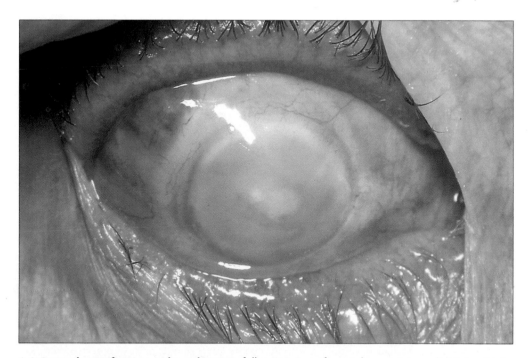

6.8 Corneal opacification without thinning, following circumferential necrotizing scleritis in which the limbal circulation had been almost completely destroyed.

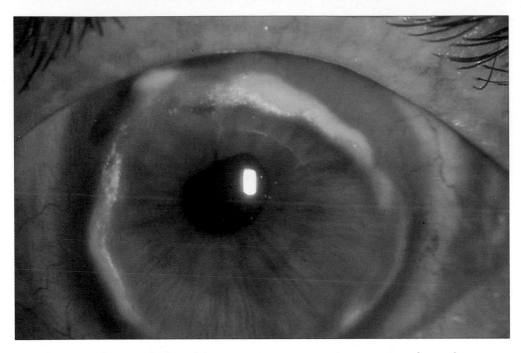

6.9 Infiltrates at the central edge of the cornea in a woman with severe circumferential recurrent necrotizing scleritis. The infiltrates increased in amount with each attack and regressed slightly in between.

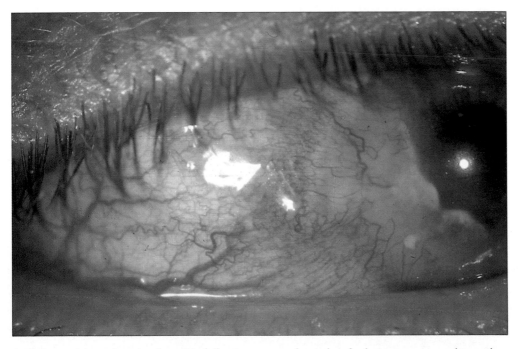

6.10 Progressive sclerosing keratitis following repeated attacks of scleritis in one quadrant. The cornea has become translucent and vascularized, with lipid deposits at the interface with normal cornea.

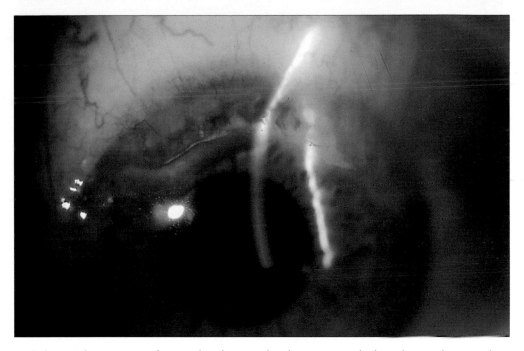

6.11 Contact lens cornea. The peripheral cornea has become entirely thin whereas the central cornea is of normal thickness.

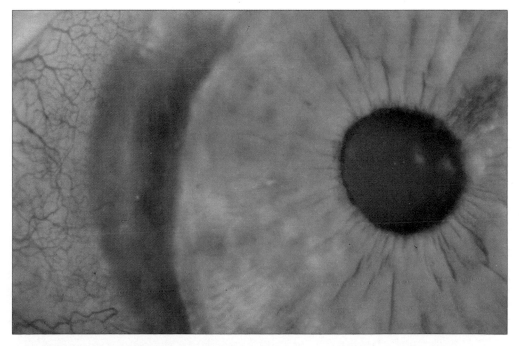

6.12 Peripheral corneal gutter which has occurred as a result of chronic low-grade scleral inflammation in the regions adjacent to the gutter. The vessels which have entered the gutter are thin and looped together, indicating inactivity and chronicity.

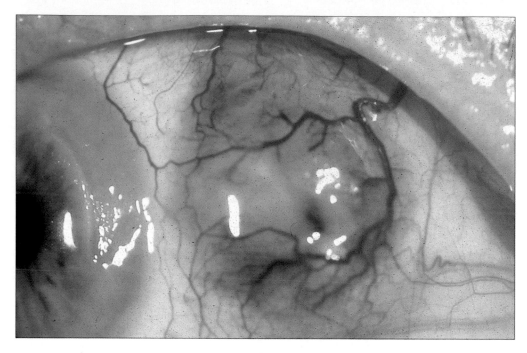

6.13 Corneal destruction adjacent to an area of necrotizing scleritis. The cornea is infiltrated but not vascularized. Large anastomatic channels surround the necrotic areas.

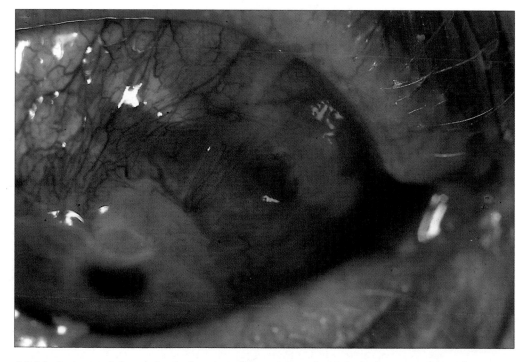

6.14 Active corneal destruction in the area of necrotizing scleritis with ulceration of the advancing edge.

6.15 Sclerokeratitis following herpes zoster infection. Although the appearances in **6.5, 6.6** are the most common seen in herpes zoster, if the response to the inflammatory stimulus is very intense, peripheral destruction of corneal tissue can arise. This sclerokeratitis, which occurred five weeks after the infection started, required systemic steroid therapy to control it.

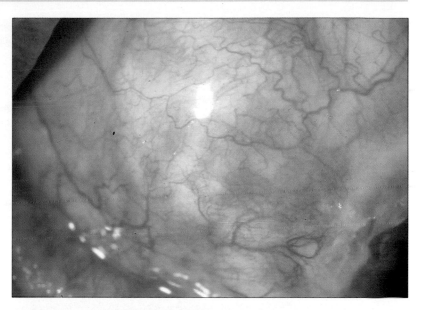

6.16, 6.17 Sclerokeratitis following herpes zoster infection. A further patient with even more severe peripheral corneal destruction one year after an attack of herpes zoster ophthalmicus. The patterns of corneal change, which are independent of the initiating cause, are the result of an immune response to the causative agent. Similar changes can be seen when the scleritis has been induced either by bacteria or other viruses or in surgically induced necrotizing scleritis (SINS).

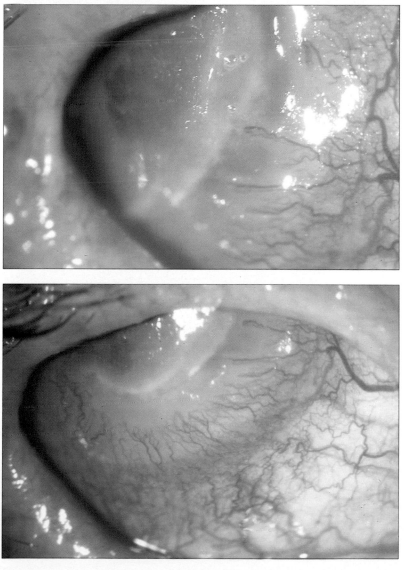

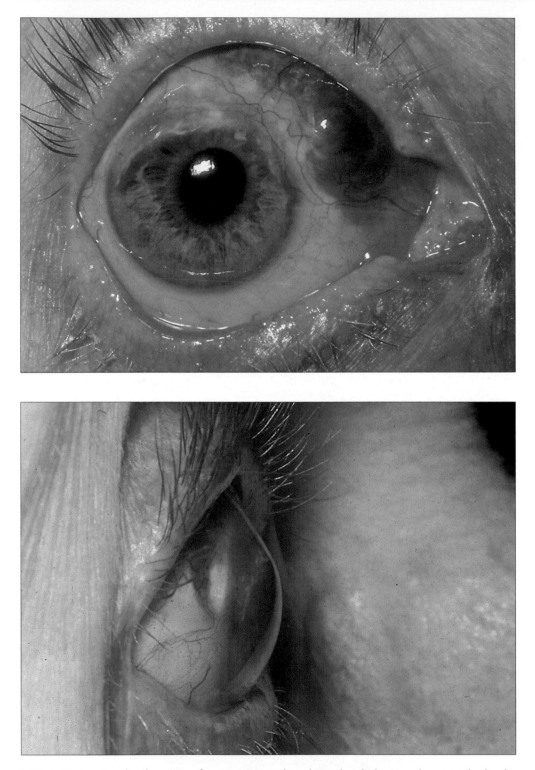

6.18, 6.19 Severe sclerokeratitis after treatment. The scleritis has led to an almost total scleral tissue loss and a staphyloma. (It is rare for staphylomas to occur unless the intraocular pressure is raised.) The upper half of the cornea is bowed forward as a result of the scleral thinning and raised intraocular pressure.

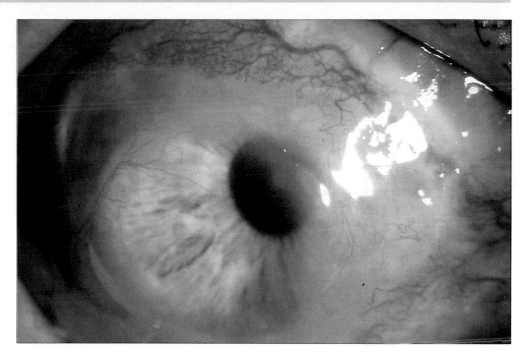

6.20 Active sclerokeratitis in necrotizing scleritis. The normal limbal architecture has disappeared and there is circumferential opacification and vascularization of the peripheral cornea. The cases in **6.1** and **6.2** would progress to this if left untreated.

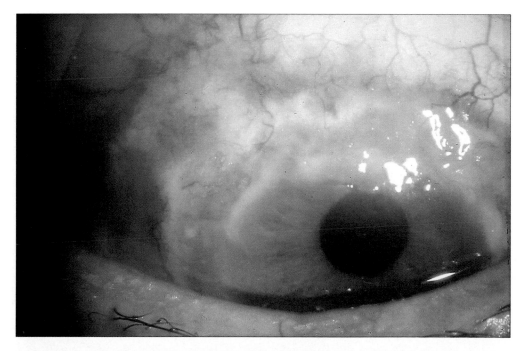

6.21 An extension of a scleral granuloma on the peripheral cornea leads to destruction of the normal limbal tissue, irregular corneal guttering and infiltration with inflammatory cells.

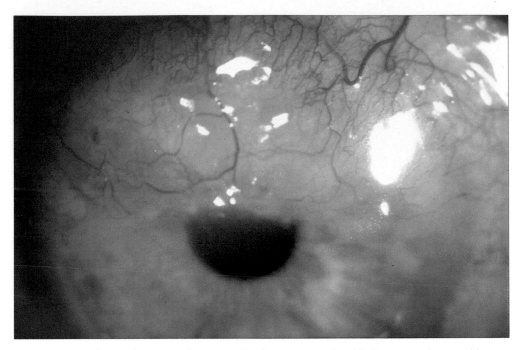

6.22 An unusual granulomatous change within the stroma and epithelium in a 65-year-old man who has had multiple attacks of sclerokeratitis in the same region over many years.

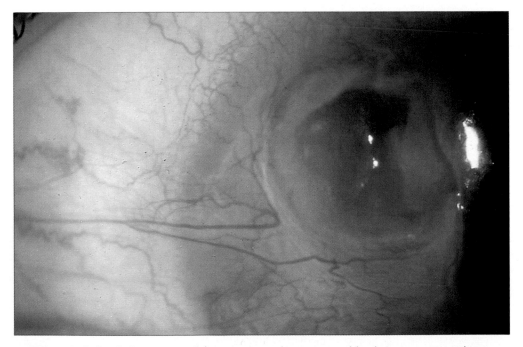

6.23 A central island of cornea is all that remains in this 35-year-old Pakistani woman with severe active rheumatoid arthritis. The patient also has Sjögren's syndrome but intensive and effective treatment of the dry eye did not alter the corneal situation although the filaments disappeared. The sclerokeratitis required immunosuppressant therapy for its control and the central area of the cornea has remained clear.

7.
Underlying Systemic Disease

Scleritis is found in patients who have some underlying autoimmune disorder. The precipitating cause in the eye is damage to the ocular tissue from mechanical, surgical, bacterial or viral trauma.

Sclerokeratitis is commonly associated with the sero-positive connective tissue disorders, usually occurring in the vasculitic phase of these diseases (**7.1–7.4**). It is therefore most commonly seen in association with: rheumatoid arthritis (**7.5–7.7**); systemic lupus erythematosus (**7.8–7.13**); and the systemic vasculitides, such as polyarteritis nodosa, Wegener's granulomatosis and relapsing polychondritis.

Rheumatoid arthritis

Although vasculitis is a constant feature of the disorders connected with scleritis and its associated corneal changes, it is by no means certain that it is the primary change in the development of the disease. The inflammatory joint changes of rheumatoid arthritis are typically seen in the early stages of the disease and if any eye signs occur at this stage they tend to involve the episclera only. The pattern only changes late in the disease, corresponding to the period in which the joint changes are quiescent and burnt out and the extra-articular manifestations of rheumatoid nodules, skin ulceration and vasculitic rash appear. At this stage, all the manifestations of sclerokeratitis, including scleromalacia perforans, become apparent; the severity depends on the intensity of the immune response.

Wegener's granulomatosis and polyarteritis nodosa

In those conditions in which vasculitis plays a prominent part in the systemic disease, such as Wegener's granulo-matosis and polyarteritis nodosa, the eye condition has a characteristic appearance. Patients usually present with an elevated irregular granuloma (**5.84–5.87, 7.14–7.17**), which if treated effectively leads to loss of tissue but not loss of integrity of the globe (**7.14–7.17**). If these granulo-matous changes are at the limbus, the peripheral corneal destructive changes transgress the limbus, affecting both cornea and sclera. This does not happen in other melting or destructive disorders where the changes remain either within the sclera or within the cornea. When associated with a systemic vasculitis, corneal gutters are always preceded by corneal infiltration deep to Bowman's membrane which disappears as soon as adequate therapy is given (**7.15–7.17**). It is important to detect this group of diseases early, because even the mildest scleritis can be associated with severe systemic disease. This is of particular importance where the renal tract is involved, as the patient may be unaware that anything is amiss until very late in the disease. The anti-nuclear cytoplasmic antibody test (ANCA) is crucial to the diagnosis of these diseases, and specific immunosuppressive therapy is now available for them. Patients require long and continued medical supervision, because even after a period of remission the disease can become reactivated and need further intensive active treatment (**7.21–7.27**).

Relapsing polychondritis

Patients with relapsing polychondritis almost always develop scleral disease during the course of their illness. Although the exact aetiology is unknown, it is assumed to be an autoimmune vasculitis associated with specific antibodies which attack cartilage, type VI collagen and similar connective tissues. When the eye is involved, the patients develop a particularly severe and intractable scleritis which can involve the anterior and posterior segments of the eye. This condition is not as uncommon as previously supposed (**7.28–7.30**).

Vasculitic lesions of the hands in a patient with rheumatoid arthritis and anterior scleritis

7.1–7.4 *The black vasculitic lesions affect the nail folds and palmar surface of the thumb. These appeared simultaneously with the area of scleritis.*

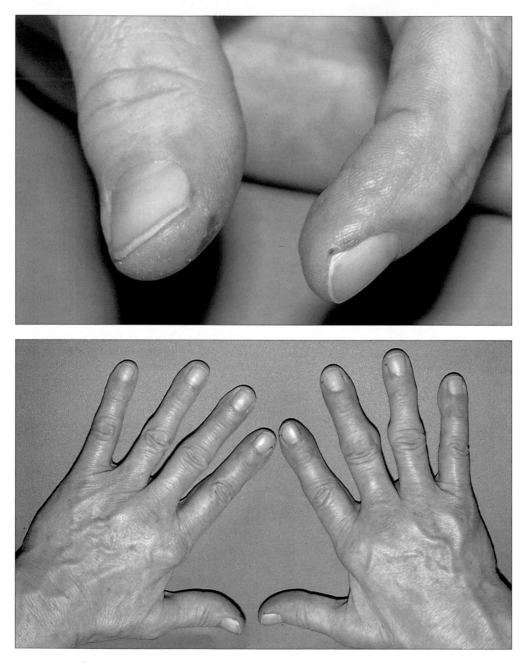

7.1, 7.2 Swelling of the metacarpo-phalangeal joints characteristic of rheumatoid arthritis.

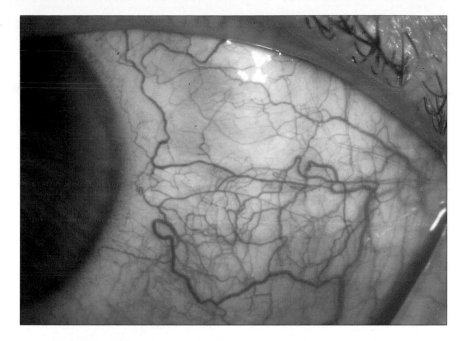

7.3 Translucency of the sclera superiorly, indicating previous attacks of scleritis. This sclera is not necessarily thin; the translucency is caused by the rearrangement of the collagen fibres during the healing process.

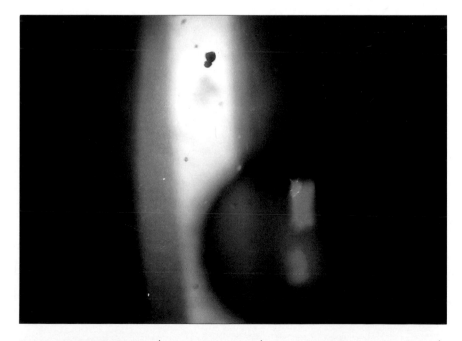

7.4 Keratic precipitates in the same patient as shown in **7.1–7.3**. Uveitis is extremely rare in patients with scleral disease. If seen, it indicates severe granulomatous disease which almost always involves the ciliary body.

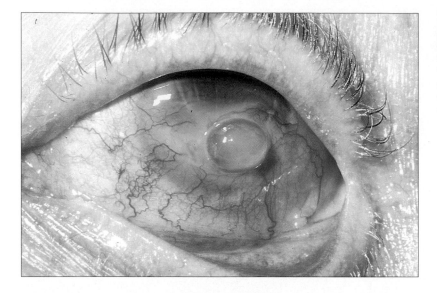

7.5 Descemetocoele formation in a patient with long-standing sclero-keratitis. In rheumatoid arthritis the changes that start in the cornea tend to remain in the cornea and those that start in the sclera stay within the scleral tissue; however, occasionally both tissues can be affected as here.

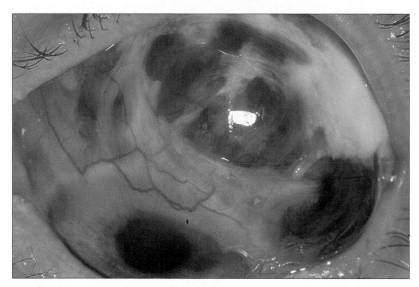

7.6, 7.7 Scleromalacia perforans. This condition occurs almost exclusively in female patients with long-standing inactive rheumatoid arthritis. The sclera becomes infarcted and resorbed. Once this has occurred very little change takes place. Ten years separate these two photographs.

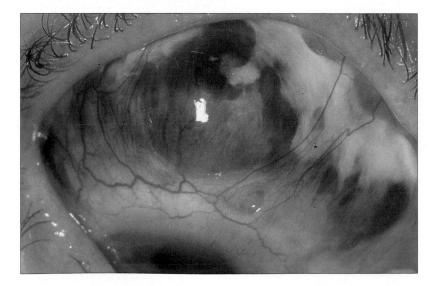

Systemic lupus erythematosus

7.8–7.13 *A 35-year-old female with sclerokeratitis. She shows the typical 'butterfly' rash over the nose and cheek (**7.8**). This is accompanied by a sclerokeratitis.*

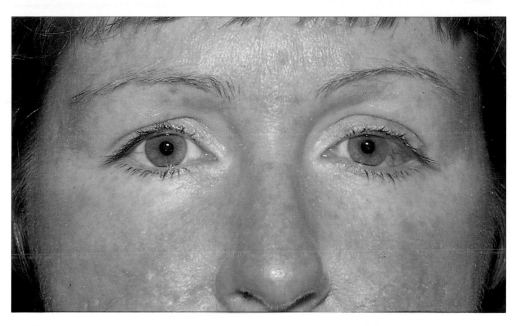

7.8 Systemic lupus erythematosus. Typical butterfly rash over the nose and cheek.

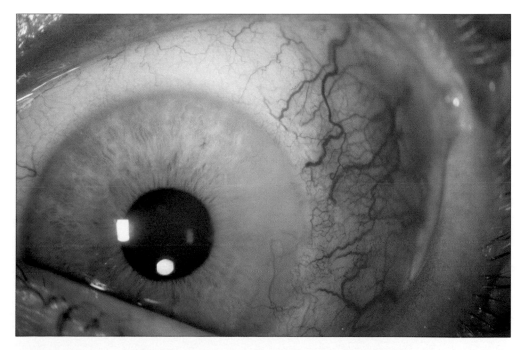

7.9 Systemic lupus erythematosus. An area of sclerokeratitis. Although the scleritis involves the eye from 1 to 5 o'clock, new vessels have only invaded the cornea between 3 and 4 o'clock. There are new vessel loops in the cornea which are active, leaking at the tips leaving a corneal haze from serum residues.

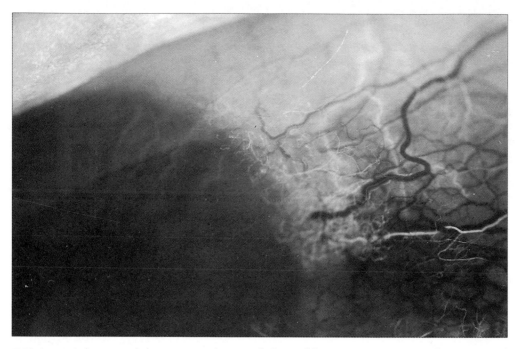

7.10 Systemic lupus erythematosus. Early arterial phase of fluorescein angiogram. There is normal arterial filling above, but almost none in the watershed zone between 2 and 3 o'clock.

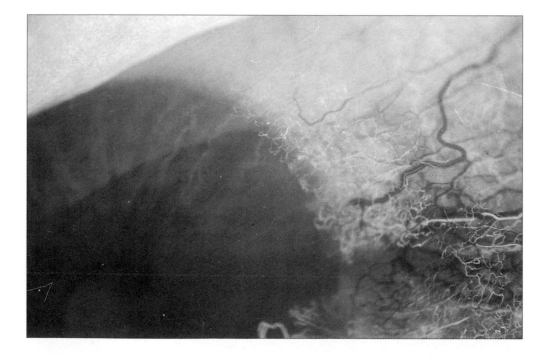

7.11 Systemic lupus erythematosus. Late venous phase of angiogram. There is grossly delayed filling of the limbal circulation adjacent to the limbus. It is in this region that the new vessels have entered the cornea.

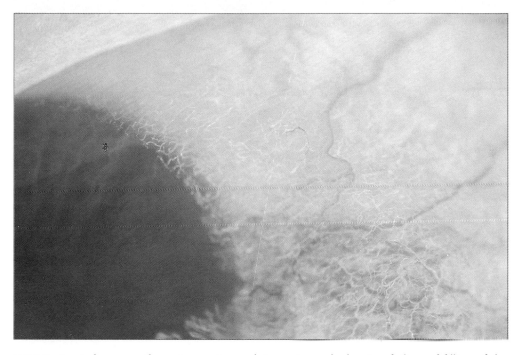

7.12 Systemic lupus erythematosus. A very late angiograph showing failure of filling of the superficial vessels at the limbus. The intra-corneal vessels are competent even though the upper ones are straight.

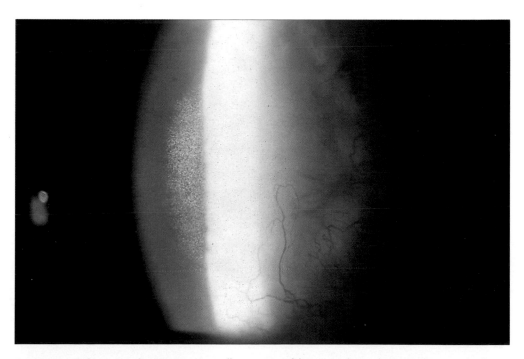

7.13 Systemic lupus erythematosus. Retroillumination of the corneal vessels (**7.9**). The vascular loops are joined, but there has been substantial leakage into the corneal stroma.

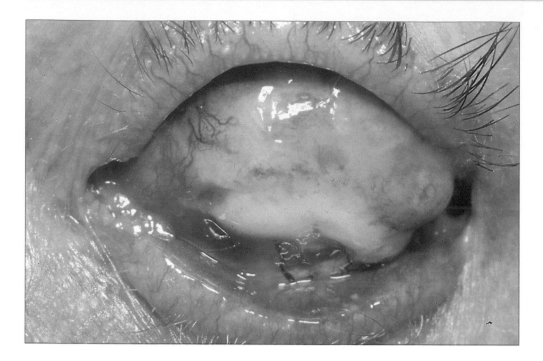

7.14 Wegener's granulomatosis. A granuloma of the limbal sclera extending into the cornea in a 60-year-old white patient; this flattened on steroid and cyclophosphamide treatment and was later successfully grafted. The patient was ANCA positive but at this stage had no other systemic manifestations of the disease. However, two years later he developed an orbital and nasal granuloma which again responded to treatment.

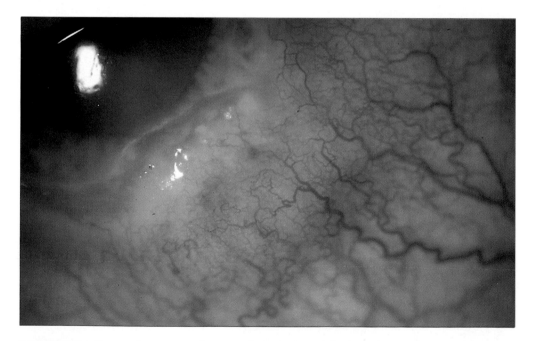

7.15 Wegener's granulomatosis. The typical appearance of a limbal granuloma in Wegener's granulomatosis and periarteritis nodosa. The grey infiltrate at the central edge of the corneal lesion is at the level of Bowman's membrane and will disappear when therapy becomes effective. This patient died from septicaemic shock originating from an infected lung lesion.

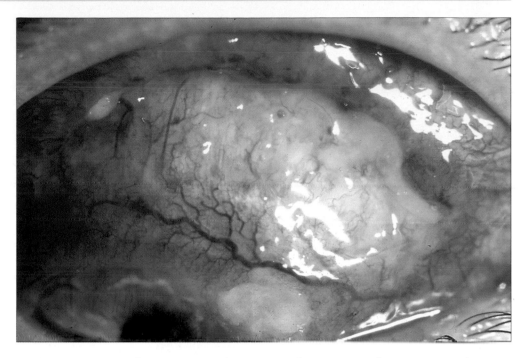

7.16 Wegener's granulomatosis. A similar patient to that in **7.14,** with a severe granulomatous sclerokeratitis. The limbus is destroyed at 1 o'clock, and there is infiltration and destruction of the limbus elsewhere.

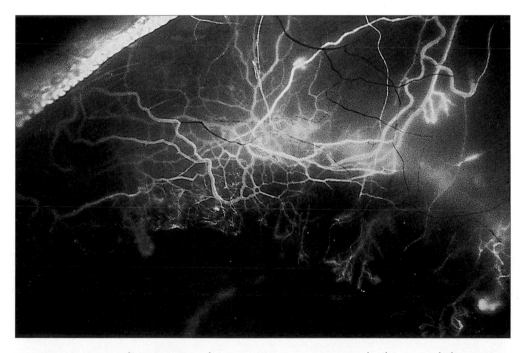

7.17 Wegener's granulomatosis. Low-dose anterior segment angiography (late arterial phase) upper outer quadrant of the patient in **7.16.** This shows very limited perfusion of the larger limbal vessels and occlusion of the superficial ones. Actively leaking new vessels are entering the cornea. There is a focal arteriolar leak in the episcleral arterial circle.

Wegener's granulomatosis

7.18–7.20 A 68-year-old white woman with biopsy-proven Wegener's granulomatosis with nasal and chest lesions, presented with an appearance similar to that in *7.14, 7.16*. After treatment with pulsed steroid and cyclophosphamide, the granuloma resolved to give this appearance.

7.18–7.20 Wegener's granulomatosis.

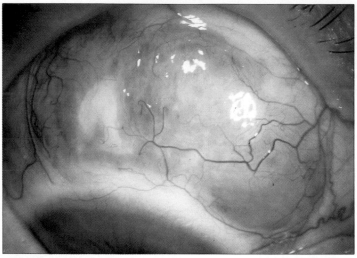

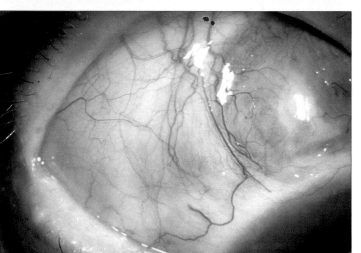

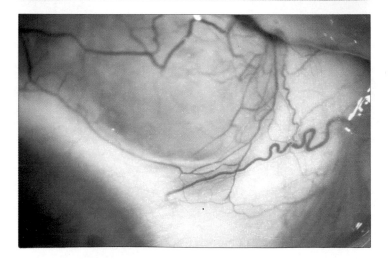

Periarteritis nodosa

7.21–7.27 This 54-year-old Indian man presented with a severely painful right eye and a severe necrotizing sclerokeratitis which was treated with systemic steroid and a cornea–sclera graft. The eye settled down and remained inactive, the graft becoming incorporated into the host tissue. Four years later, during an acute exacerbation of the systemic disease, the left eye became red and painful. He was found to have an anterior and posterior scleritis and a retinoschisis. The patient had an intense sclerokeratitis largely confined to the limbal area with corneal infiltration and distortion of limbal blood vessels. Anterior segment fluorescein angiography showed an extremely slow circulation, very narrow arteries, very dilated veins and almost absent filling of the episcleral circulation. The limbal arcades, which are largely supplied by the conjunctival vessels, are broken and leak dye.

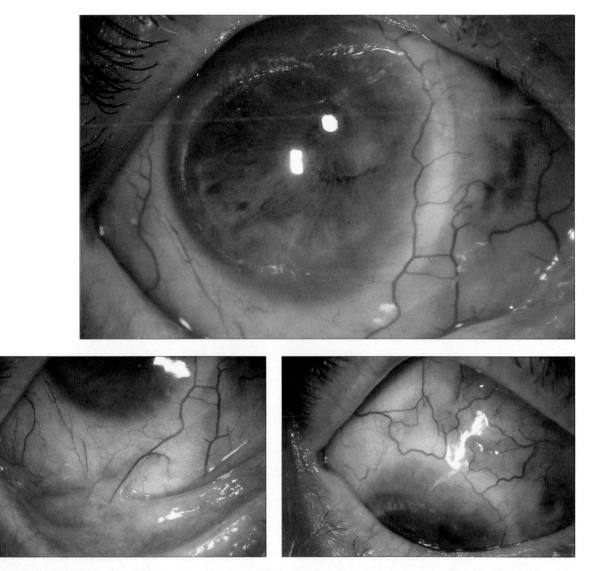

7.21–7.23 Right eye four years after corneo-scleral transplantation for acute necrotizing sclerokeratitis. The graft is now entirely incorporated into host tissue.

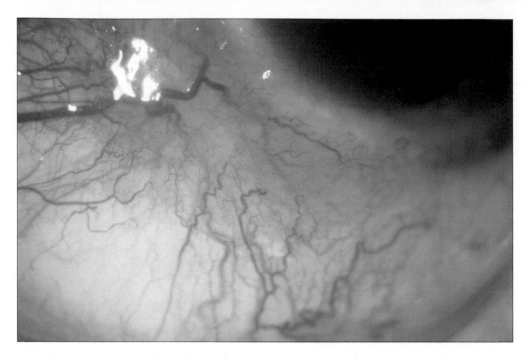

7.24 Clinical appearance of the left eye. There is an intense, active scleritis superiorly. The angiogram is taken at the junction between the obviously inflamed tissue and the apparently normal tissue. Note that even in this region the vascular pattern is abnormal and the limbal vasculature disturbed.

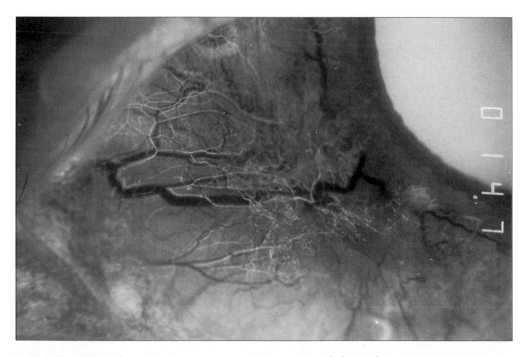

7.25 Periarteritis nodosa. Anterior segment angiogram. Arterial phase. The arteries are very narrow and slow to fill.

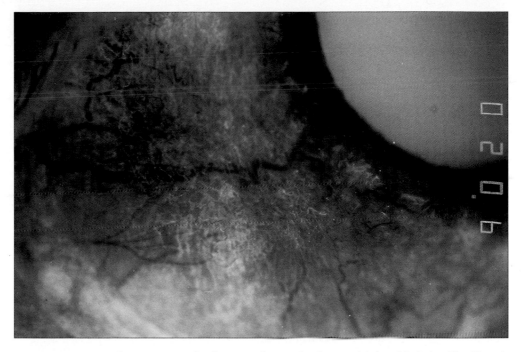

7.26 Periarteritis nodosa. Six seconds after **7.25**, the episcleral network has still failed to fill. Although obviously full of blood (**7.24**), the large vessel filling is not seen, possibly because of a thickened vascular wall or sluggish flow.

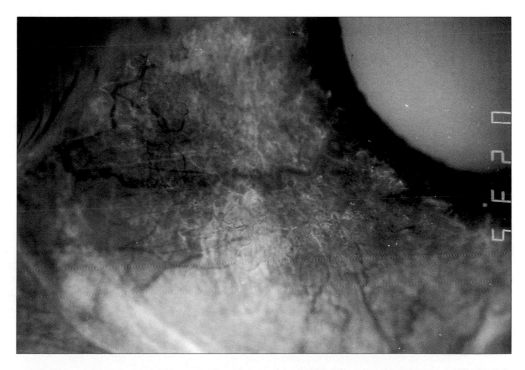

7.27 Periarteritis nodosa. Late venous phase. The episcleral network remains unfilled. The conjunctival vessels supply the limbus. These vessels leak at their tips.

Anterior and posterior scleritis in relapsing polychondritis

7.28–7.30 This 65-year-old white woman presented with a gradual onset of a painful red eye and reduction of vision. She had a sclerokeratitis and a large posterior scleral nodule seen on ultrasonography *(7.30)*. The retina and choroid were also totally detached. She had not thought the loss of the nose tip or alteration in her voice to be important. In this instance it was not painful.

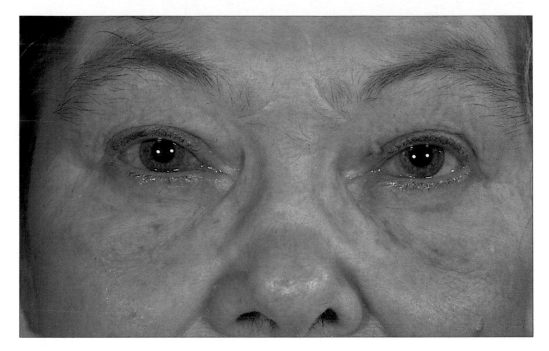

7.28 Relapsing polychondritis. The loss of the cartilage at the tip of the nose in a patient with relapsing polychondritis and a severe sclerokeratitis.

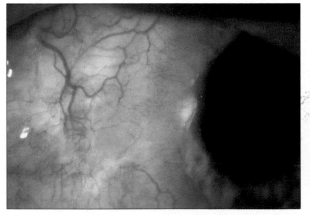

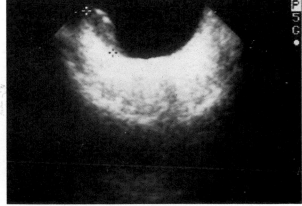

7.29 Relapsing polychondritis. Active sclerokeratitis in the left eye. Scleritis in this condition is extremely resistant to treatment and almost always requires the use of combined steroid and immunosuppressive therapy.

7.30 Relapsing polychondritis. Scleral and choroidal swelling in the left eye. The right eye had an exudative retinal detachment.

Other associated systemic diseases

Uveitis and scleritis are almost mutually exclusive conditions. If cells are found in the anterior or posterior chambers in patients with scleritis this indicates either that they have severe disease involving the ciliary body or that they have mixed connective tissue disease. It is well known that Crohn's disease and ulcerative colitis have joint manifestations, and if there is eye involvement this takes the form of an acute anterior uveitis. However, some patients with these conditions will present with a scleritis indistinguishable from those seen with the seropositive arthritides (**7.31–7.43**) whilst others present with a migratory scleral, corneal or episcleral disease very similar to conjunctival phlyctenular disease (**7.44–7.58**).

Sclerokeratitis in mixed connective tissue disease

7.31–7.43 This 66-year-old white man had had ulcerative colitis for 6 years. Four years after the onset, he developed scleritis which required pulsed cyclophosphamide and prednisolone for its control. He also developed a pyodermic granuloma of the leg six months before presentation when he was found to have a mild scleritis and a rapidly advancing peripheral corneal gutter.

7.31

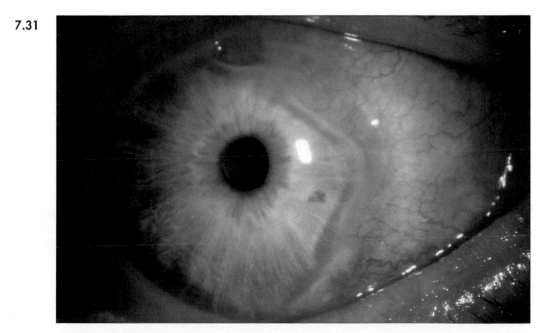

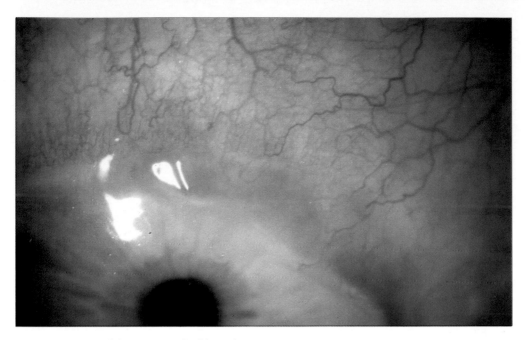

7.32 Upper part of the gutter and infiltrated cornea.

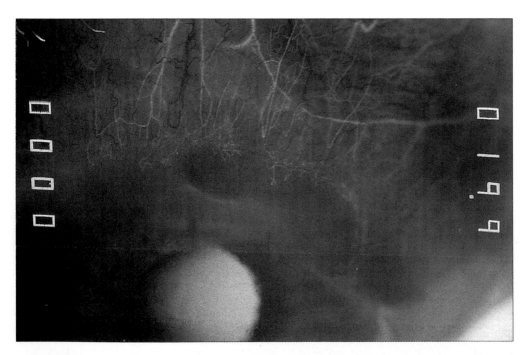

7.33 Anterior segment fluorescein angiogram. Late arterial phase. There is an immediate and rapid filling of the limbal vasculature in the region of the corneal gutter.

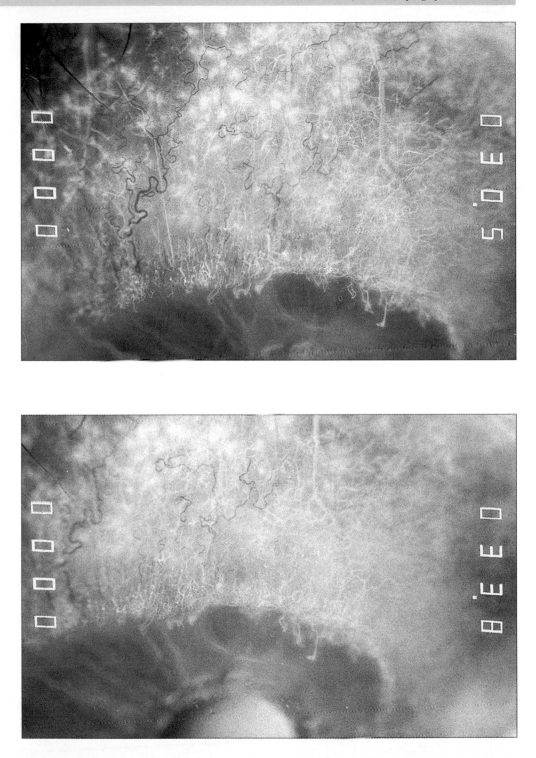

7.34, 7.35 Late venous phase. New vessels are entering the base of the gutter and surrounding its advancing edge. There is also leakage from the episcleral vessels at the limbus. Filling is delayed in the apparently unaffected region at 12 o'clock, which also affects the iris vessels in this segment. This is not necessarily abnormal, but note that the limbal arcade is disrupted in this region.

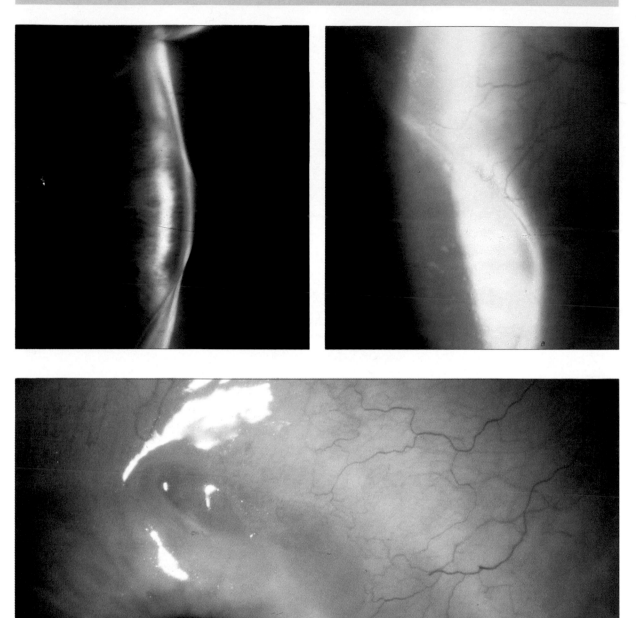

7.36–7.38 Three months later, following treatment, there has been no advance of the ulcer although the cornea is still oedematous. The limbal vessels have re-joined and are not leaking, indicating inactivity.

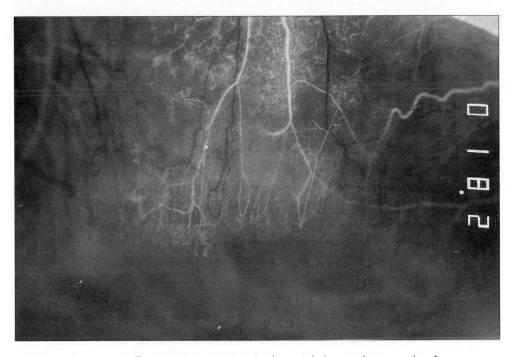

7.39 Anterior segment fluorescein angiogram (mid-arterial phase). Three months after treatment the area above the tip of the gutter still shows slight early leakage, but elsewhere the filling pattern is normal.

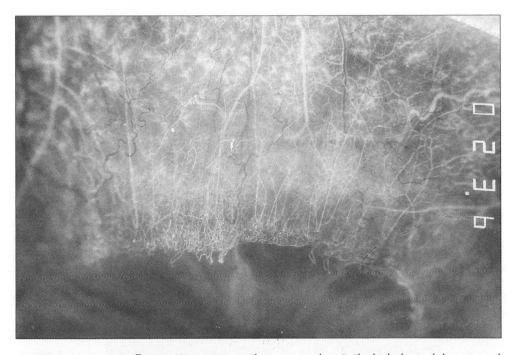

7.40 Anterior segment fluorescein angiogram (late-venous phase). The limbal vessels have joined at their tips and no longer leak.

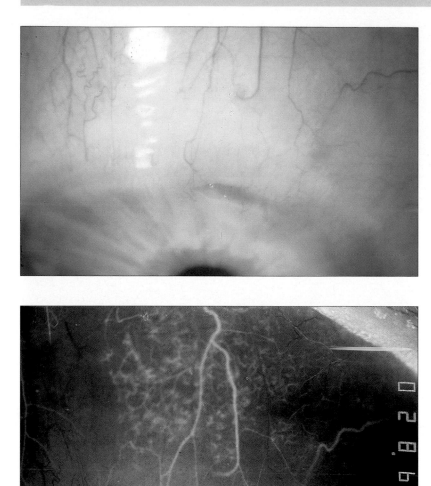

7.41 Two years later the ulcer is still visible but obviously inactive. The blood supply at the limbus is unchanged although the vessels adjacent to the gutter are no longer dilated.

7.42 Arterial segment fluorescein angiogram (mid-arterial phase). A normal filling pattern has been restored.

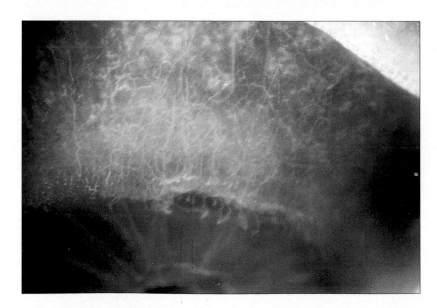

7.43 Arterial segment fluorescein angiogram (late-venous phase). The vascular pattern is identical to that in **7.40** showing that new vessels, once established, are permanent. Remodelling does not occur. Note that the iris is now also normally perfused (cf. **7.34**).

Migratory 'phylctenular' sclerokeratitis in mixed connective tissue disease

7.44–7.56 This 41-year-old white woman had a 6-year history of Crohn's disease, erythema nodosa and an arthropathy including pain in temporo-mandibular and metacarpo-phalangeal joints for which she was on 10 mg daily prednisolone and 100 mg of azathioprine. She presented with a severely painful eye with a scleral nodule and corneal infiltrate. This was satisfactorily treated by temporarily increasing the dose of steroids. The angiographic appearances shown in the following sequences are in marked contrast to those seen in necrotizing scleritis.

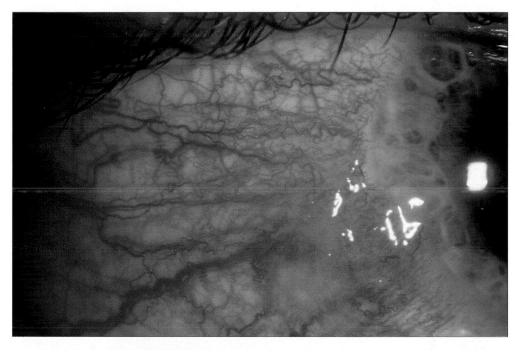

7.44 Migratory 'phylctenular' sclerokeratitis. The clinical appearance at presentation. The sclera appeared to be swollen under the conjunctival lesion.

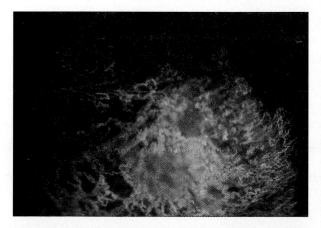

7.45 Migratory 'phylctenular' sclerokeratitis. Mid-arterial phase of anterior segment flourescein angiogram reveals that the lesion is confined to the conjunctiva.

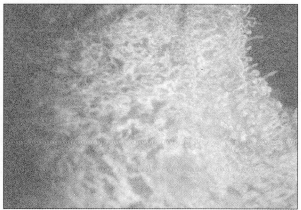

7.46 Migratory 'phylctenular' sclerokeratitis. Late-venous phase. An intense limbal inflammation. A few new deep and straight active vessels can be seen.

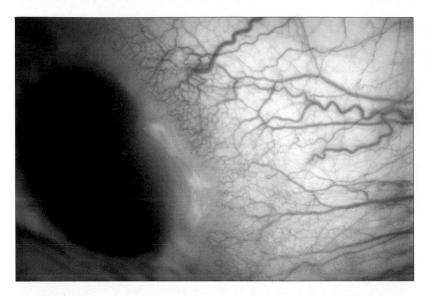

7.47 Migratory 'phylctenular' sclero-keratitis. Four years later she presented again with purely corneal lesions. The limbal vessels were very congested but there was no vascular abnormality.

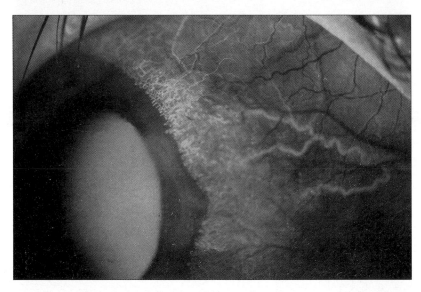

7.48 Migratory 'phylctenular' sclero-keratitis. Low-dose anterior segment flourescein angiogram (mid-arterial phase). Note that in spite of the limbal infiltration, there is no abnormality of the limbal arcades.

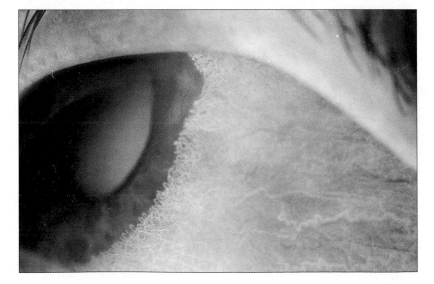

7.49 Migratory 'phylctenular' sclero-keratitis. Late-venous phase. A normal filling pattern is seen.

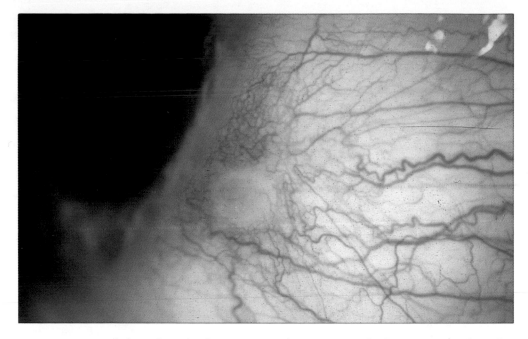

7.50 Migratory 'phylctenular' sclerokeratitis. Over the next six months she presented with similar lesions at the limbus in different anomaly locations. One of these lesions stained with fluorescein and none left any vascular when the lesion resolved.

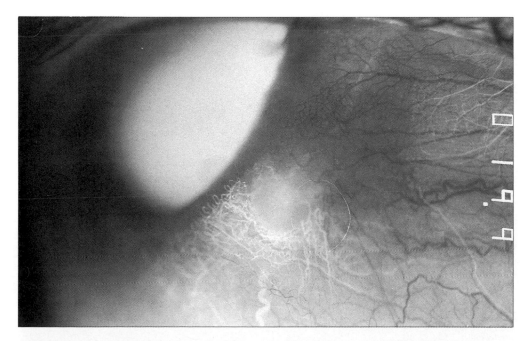

7.51 Migratory 'phylctenular' sclerokeratitis. Low-dose anterior segment flourescein angiogram (arterial phase). There is no filling of the conjunctiva over the lesion, but elsewhere the pattern is normal.

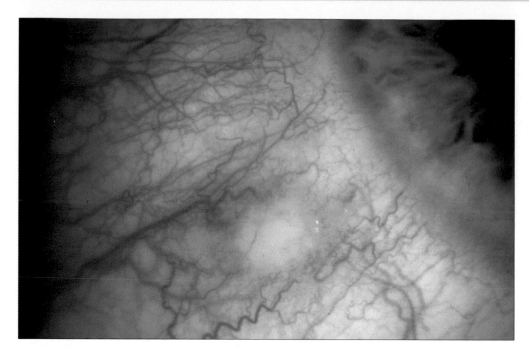

7.52 Migratory 'phylctenular' sclerokeratitis. Another very similar lesion which appeared suddenly and very painfully 4 months later.

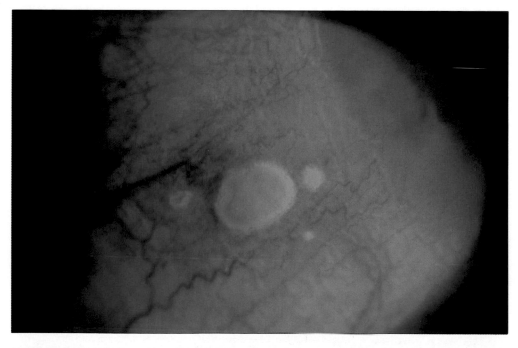

7.53 Migratory 'phylctenular' sclerokeratitis. Infra-red photograph of the lesion in **7.52** confirming its superficial nature.

7.54 Migratory 'phylctenular' sclero-keratitis. This was the final lesion to affect this lady. She has been followed up for 8 years and has had no recurrences.

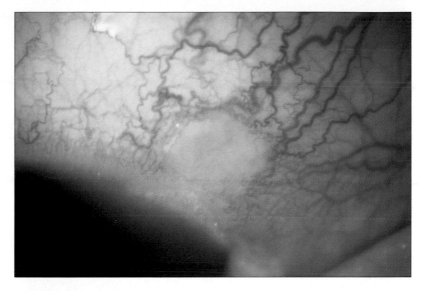

7.55, 7.56 Migratory 'phylctenular' sclerokeratitis. Low-dose anterior segment flourescein angiogram (mid arterial **7.55**, late venous **7.56**). These again show the superficial nature of the lesion and the lack of disturbance of the normal circulation and blood vessels.

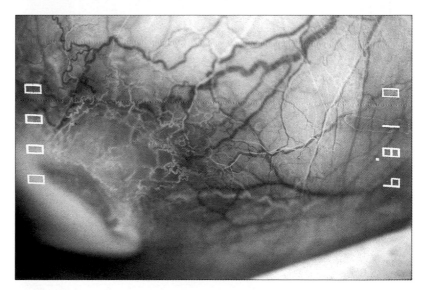

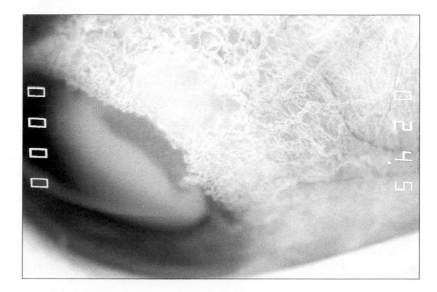

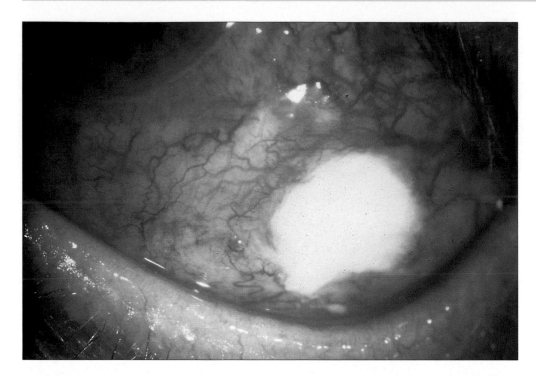

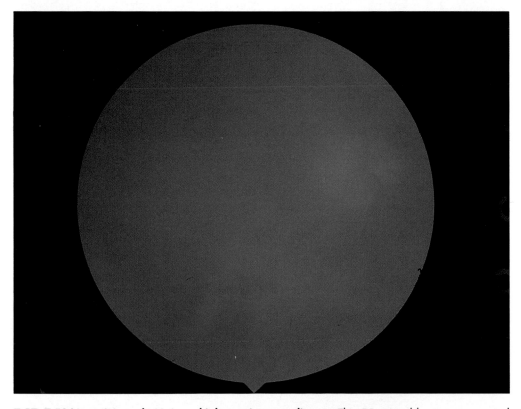

7.57, 7.58 Necrotizing scleritis in multiple autoimmune disease. This 55-year-old woman presented with a necrotizing scleritis in her only good eye. She had developed dysthyroid ophthalmopathy 25 years earlier and had lost her other eye despite treatment and orbital decompression. Shortly after this she developed diabetes with retinopathy which became proliferative. Three years before she presented with scleritis, she had also developed typical rheumatoid arthritis.

8.
Surgically Induced Scleritis

Apart from the pathological and serological findings, there is good clinical evidence that scleritis is an autoimmune disorder. Quite apart from its appearance in patients who have single or multiple autoimmune disorders (**7.57, 7.58**), there is a group of patients, who may or may not show surgical evidence of connective tissue disorders, who develop a particularly severe and intractable form of diffuse anterior or necrotizing scleritis when they have an eye operation. The acronym SINS (surgically induced necrotizing scleritis) has been used for this not uncommon problem. This can follow ocular surgery of any kind, including cataract, glaucoma, strabismus, and retinal detachment (**8.1–8.12**). Although the latent period from surgery to the onset of scleritis varies from the first postoperative day in a previously sensitized patient to 40 years, the commonest story is of a patient whose eye does not completely settle after surgery and after 3–4 months the eye gradually becomes more red and painful and is not helped by local medication. Some patients have had squint surgery in childhood and have responded to cataract extraction by developing a scleritis at the site of the original squint surgery.

8.1 Scleritis following trabeculectomy. The scleritis commenced three months after uncomplicated trabeculectomy. It was rapidly progressive and required intensive systemic therapy for its control.

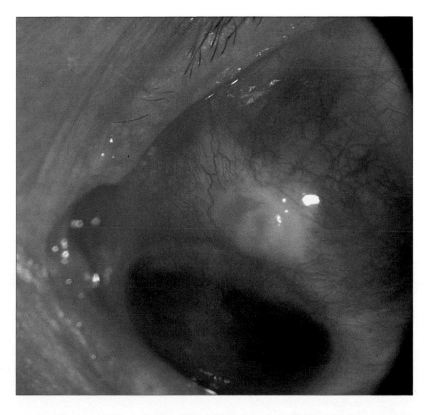

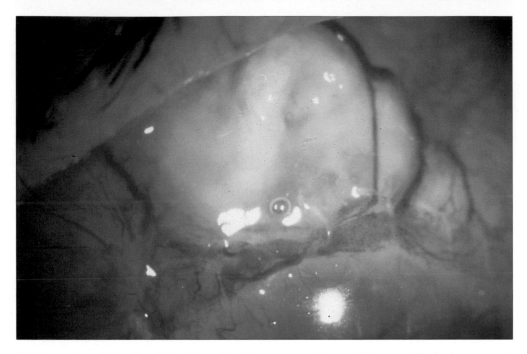

8.2 Destruction of the sclera following trabeculectomy in a 56-year-old woman. She had no systemic disease. The eye remained red following surgery, in spite of local steroid therapy. The necrotic phase started two months after surgery.

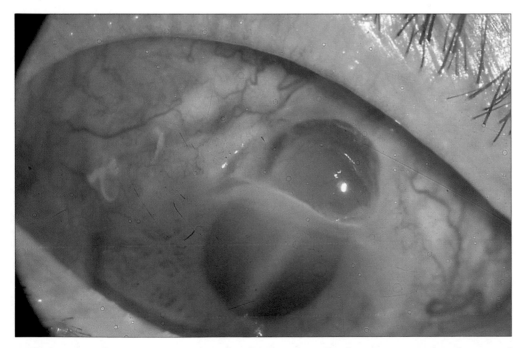

8.3 Corneal perforation in a patient who developed a sclerokeratitis six weeks after retinal detachment surgery.

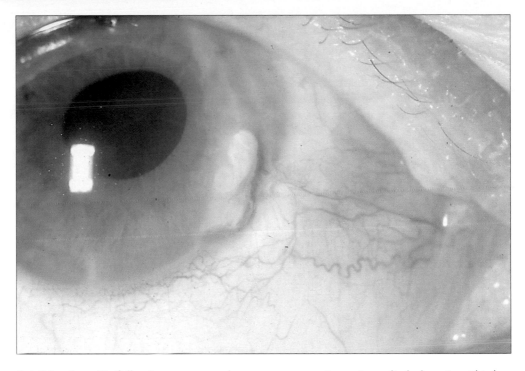

8.4 Sclerokeratitis following extracapsular cataract extraction using a limbal section. This has responded to treatment with systemic steroid.

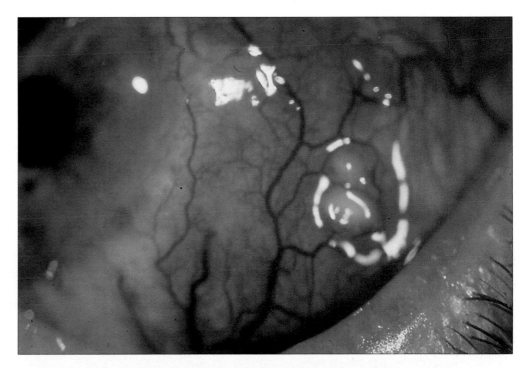

8.5 Severe scleritis developing at the site of squint surgery performed 23 years earlier.

Surgically induced necrotizing scleritis following strabismus surgery (SINS)

8.6–8.12 *This 53-year-old woman presented 10 days after an operation on her medial rectus with an apparently typical anterior scleritis superiorly away from the site of surgery. She was treated with local steroids only and the condition regressed over a period of 2 months.*

Five years later she re-presented with a necrotic lesion at the site of surgery and a diffuse scleral swelling elsewhere. An angiogram performed at that time reveals capillary non-perfusion even away from the site of necrosis. This area persists throughout the angiogram.

8.6

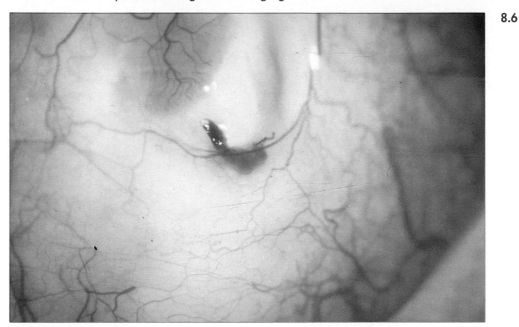

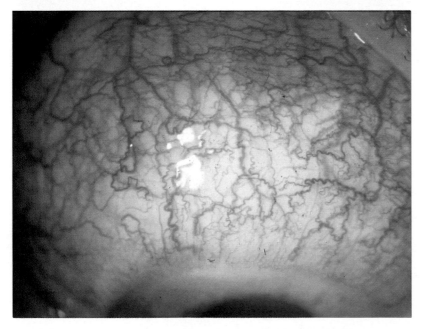

8.7 Diffuse anterior scleritis ten days after an operation on medical rectus.

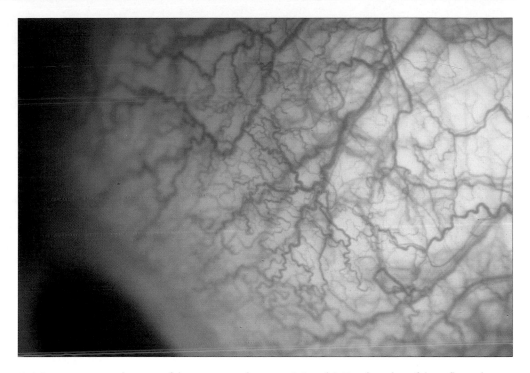

8.8 Supero-temporal region of the same eye shown in **8.6** and **8.7** at the edge of the inflamed area.

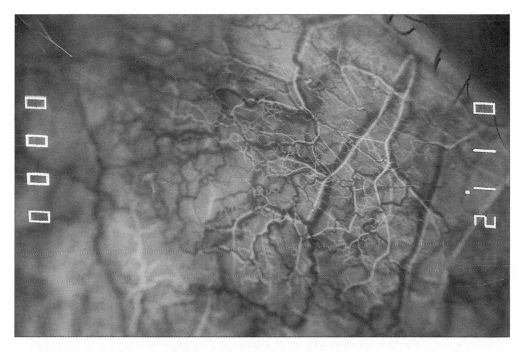

8.9 Low-dose anterior segment fluorescein angiogram (early-arterial phase). The anterior ciliary and perforating arteries fill rapidly.

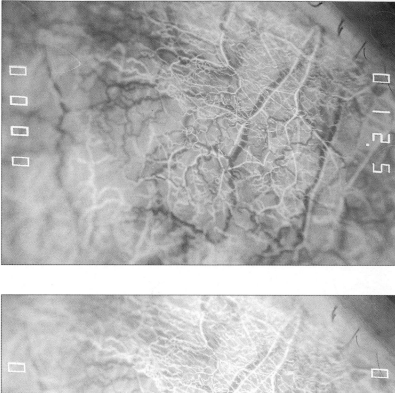

8.10 (mid-arterial phase), 8.11 (late-arterial phase), 8.12 (early-venous phase). Although the perforating arteries have filled early, the only capillary circulation seen here is from the conjuctival vessels, elsewhere there is much delayed flow.

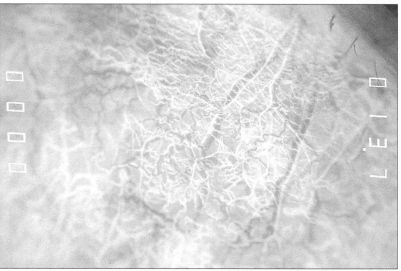

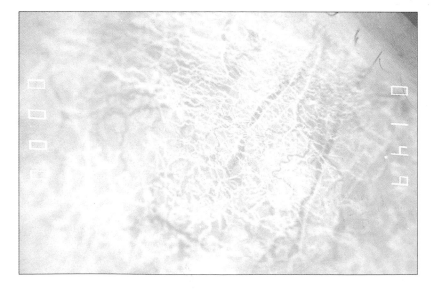

9.
Other Affections of the Sclera

Whilst almost all the acute inflammatory diseases affect the sclera or episclera, there are other conditions which can affect this tissue.

Infections

Infection of the sclera is rare partly because the scleral fibres are tightly bound together and the tissue itself has no blood supply. This is the reason why in the pre-antibiotic era, evisceration was recommended for endophthalmitis. However, infection can occur, especially in an immunosuppressed or immunodeficient patient,

either from a blood-borne infection or from a localized abscess in the tissues on either side, such as an infected scleral plomb following retinal detachment surgery.

All scleral abscesses present in a similar manner. There is an appearance of a localized tender swelling on the globe; the conjunctiva and episclera are extremely congested, but unlike scleritis the pain does not radiate to the face in the early stages of the disease. Untreated or inappropriately treated, the abscess can extend into the cornea (9.1–9.4); into the eye to give an endophthalmitis; or into the orbit to create an orbital abscess.

The common infective organisms involved are *Staphylococcus aureus, pneumococcus, Pseudomonas pyocyanea,* various fungi and Acanthamoeba. Treatment of all the conditions they cause is difficult and uncertain.

Fungal infection of the sclera

9.1–9.4 This 70-year-old Greek man presented with a very painful eye. There was intense congestion of the conjunctiva and episclera. The sclera was swollen and the deep corneal stroma adjacent to the limbus was infiltrated in one area. He was treated with systemic steroid on the assumption that there was a severe nodular scleritis. Within 5 days the corneal stromal infiltrate increased enormously, so a segmental corneal graft was performed. The organism recovered from the graft was Paecilomyces. The eye eventually recovered after a prolonged course of the appropriate antifungal agents.

9.1 Appearance of the sclera at presentation. The sclera is swollen in this area.

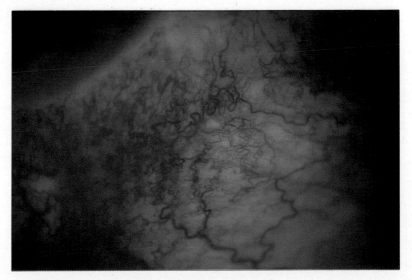

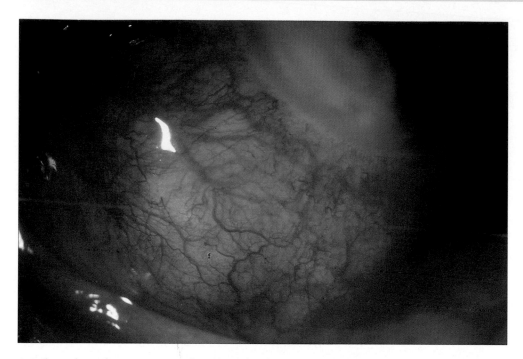

9.2 Three days after presentation the cornea has become infiltrated.

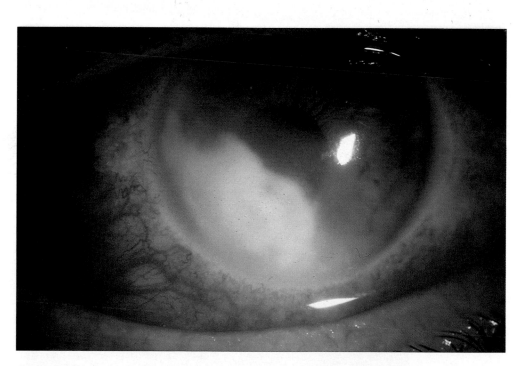

9.3 Five days after presentation. Rapid extension of the corneal infiltrate with abscess formation.

9.4 One week after segmental corneal grafting and antifungal therapy.

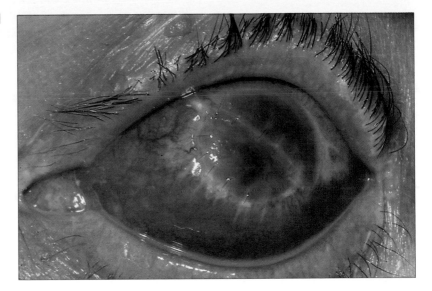

Granulomatous lesions

Granulomas occasionally occur as a result of foreign bodies, such as bamboo and grass, being embedded in the cornea. However, they are most commonly seen as part of ophthalmia nodosa (**9.5**) in which the hairs of the various varieties of hairy caterpillar become embedded in the eye. Because of the shape of the spine of the hair it will migrate inwards into the eye exciting a granulomatous reaction *en route*.

9.5 Scleral granuloma (ophthalmia nodosa). An intense inflammatory reaction, limbal granuloma and corneal opacification caused by the hairs of the hairy caterpillar of *Macrothylacia rubi* (fox moth).

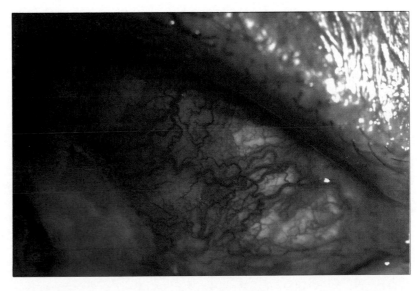

Tumours

Primary tumours of the sclera itself do not exist, but tumours may be derived from the coats which cover the sclera or the vessels and arteries which trangress it. Vascular, pigmented or florid epithelial tumours never cause confusion with inflammatory disease, but occasionally the non-pigmented naevus (**9.6**) and the dermoid cyst (**9.7**) can be mistaken for scleral inflammation. However, lymphomatous infiltration of the conjunctiva and episclera is commonly thought to be the result of an inflammation rather than an infiltration of the tissue. Lymphomas do not induce an inflammatory response (**9.8**). This together with their unusual colour differentiates them from a scleritis.

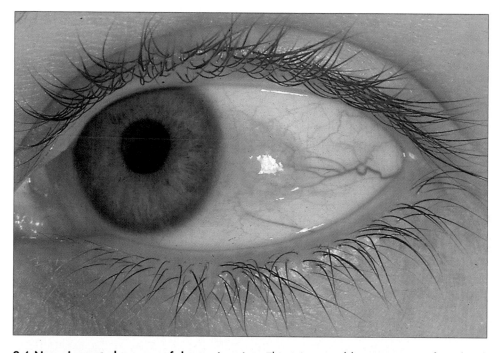

9.6 Non-pigmented naevus of the conjunctiva. This 19-year-old patient was referred with possible episcleritis. There is no inflammatory response. The lesion is well defined, a different colour to the adjacent episclera and has been present for several years.

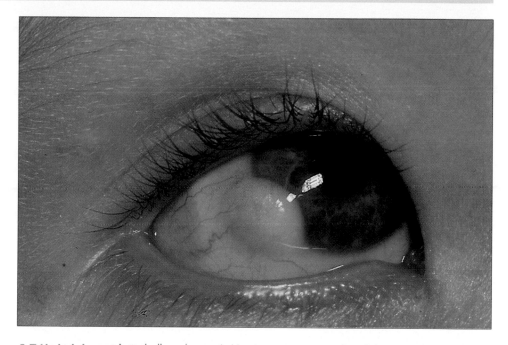

9.7 Limbal dermoid. Epibulbar dermoids like this are common, but if they are confined to the episcleral tissue they can cause confusion with inflammatory scleral disease. The mass is always raised and fixed with a fleshy pink appearance, often in the lower temporal quadrant and never invoking an inflammatory response. Careful examination reveals small hairs on the surface.

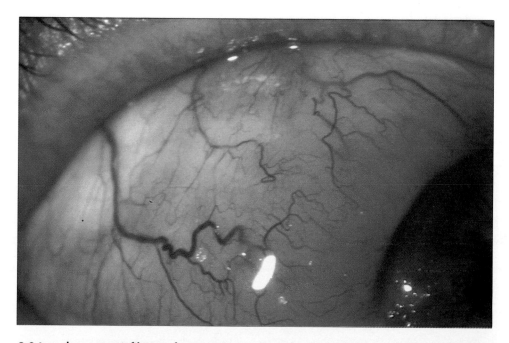

9.8 Lymphomatous infiltrate of conjunctiva and episclera. Lymphomatous infiltrates are often mistaken for episcleritis. They only induce mild discomfort and no inflammatory reaction. The colour is always different from the surrounding episclera, from which it is sharply demarcated.

Scleral hyaline plaque

Scleral hyaline plaques develops in elderly people between the cornea and the insertion of the lateral and medial rectus muscles, presumably as a result of changes in the collagen from the pulling of the intraocular muscles (**9.9, 9.10**). These plaques are solid and can occasionally become displaced, cutting through the conjunctiva and exciting an inflammatory response. Normally they should not be touched as they extend through the full thickness of the sclera and will lead to a scleral deficit if removed.

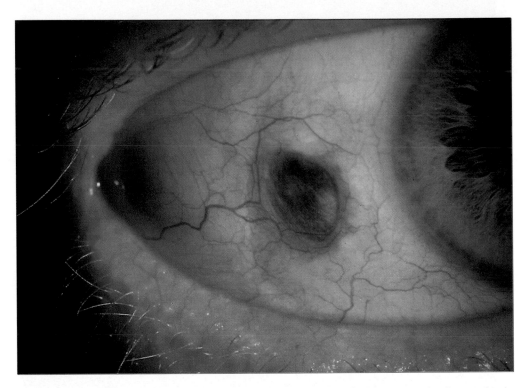

9.9 Scleral hyaline plaques. This 78-year-old woman presented with pain and a foreign-body sensation in her right eye. A 'foreign body' (the hyaline plaque) adjacent to the limbus was excised leaving a large defect in the sclera.

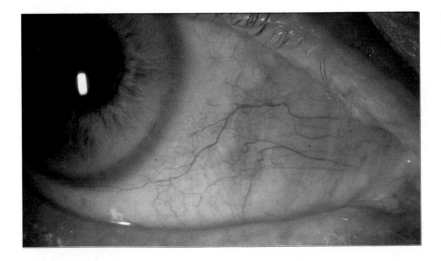

9.10 Scleral hyaline plaques. Same patient as in **9.9**. The other eye, which shows a typical hyaline plaque.

Mooren's ulceration

The most difficult differential diagnosis from sclero-keratitis is that of Mooren's ulcer. Mooren's ulcer is a purely corneal disease, whether it be of the bilateral type seen in Africans or the unilateral variety commonly seen in the Caucasian population. It is never associated with a scleritis. The limbus may be intensely congested but the inflammatory response does not extend backwards into the sclera nor is the sclera itself involved in any destructive process. It is not associated with any systemic disease. The ulcer starts about 2 mm from the limbus. The cornea becomes thickened, infiltrated and eventually guttered. The process spreads both peripherally and centrally in the cornea and once initiated may become multi-focal.

There is always infiltration of the advancing edge of the ulcer to which new vessels will grow and which is extensively undermined.

Even though it appears normal, the rest of the cornea is thickened and soft throughout. As the ulcer progresses it leaves behind thin vascularized tissue consisting of the deep layers of the cornea and Descemet's membrane covered by a thin sheet of vascularized tissue. Perforation is surprisingly uncommon, but the cornea is very vulnerable to minor trauma (**9.11–9.18**). This is unlike the peripheral ulceration of the connective tissue disorders, in which, apart from the presence of other systemic problems, the ulcer extends circumferentially rather than centrally. The peripheral corneal melting seen in the vasculitis of connective tissue disease is often accompanied by scleral inflammation and vascular occlusive changes, and perforation is more common.

Mooren's ulcer

9.11–9.18 *This diabetic Arab had a 3-year history of discomfort in the right eye but with very little inflammation. Three weeks before presentation the eye had become intensely painful. When examined he was found to have a peripheral corneal ulcer extending from 6 o'clock to 3 o'clock with a perforation of the cornea at 12 o'clock.*

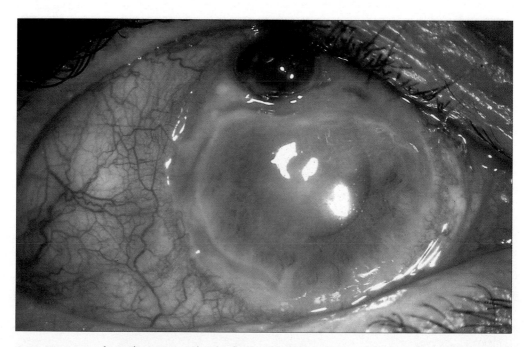

9.11 Mooren's ulcer. There is no scleral inflammation although the limbus is inflamed adjacent to the perforation. The ulcer is undermined centrally and yellow/white stromal infiltrates precede the advancing gutter centrally and circumferentially.

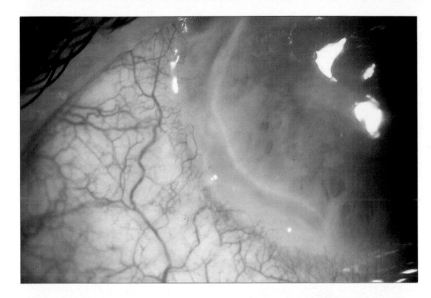

9.12 Mooren's ulcer. The cornea is swollen in the upper two-thirds of its area. There is no detectable systemic disease.

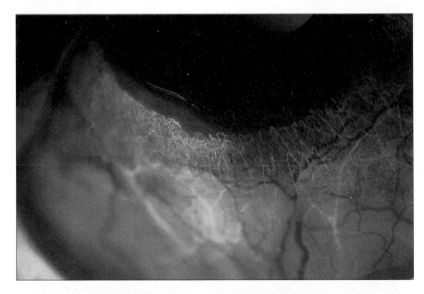

9.13 Mooren's ulcer. Anterior segment fluorescein angiogram at the advancing edge of the corneal gutter. Mid-arterial phase. Although the vessels related to the gutter are dilated, the vascular pattern is undisturbed.

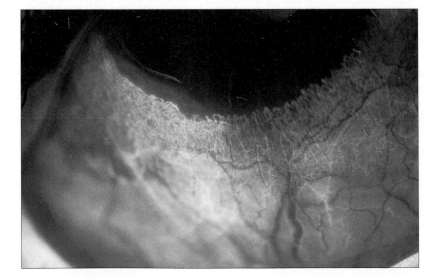

9.14 Mooren's ulcer. Venous phase. The normal vascular limbal architecture is maintained, a sharp contrast to the changes seen in sclerokeratitis.

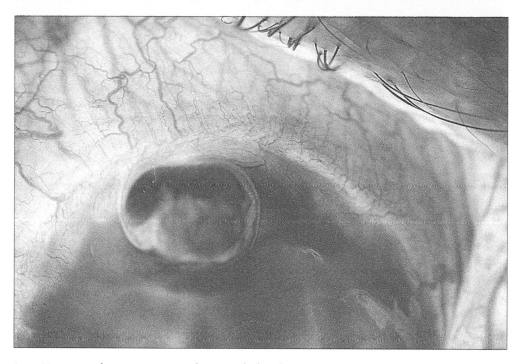

9.15 Mooren's ulcer. Late venous phase. Limbal archetecture remains almost normal even in the perforation.

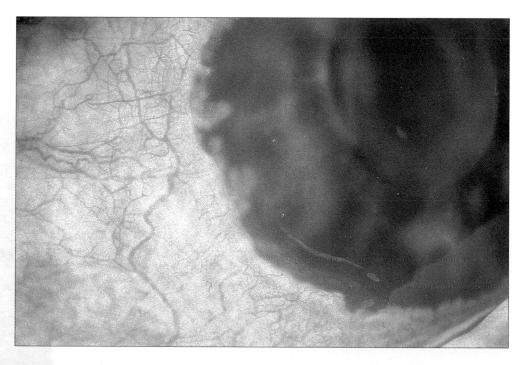

9.16 Mooren's ulcer. Late venous phase. This reveals that the vessels lying in the base of the ulcer are derived from the deep scleral plexus of vessels.

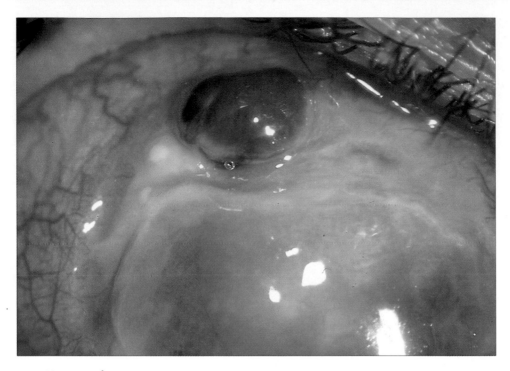

9.17 Mooren's ulcer.

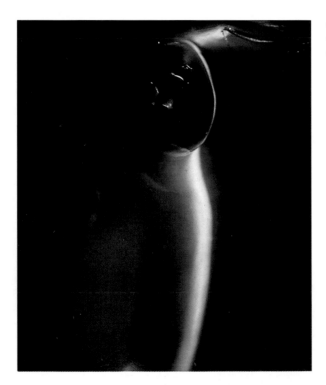

9.18 Mooren's ulcer. Detail of **9.11** to show the extreme thinning of the peripheral cornea. The infiltration is typical of the type of guttering seen in Mooren's ulceration.

Index

Figures in **bold** refer to illustrations